Alessandra Russo
Francisco B. Assumpção

Psychiatric comorbidities

Alessandra Russo
Francisco B. Assumpção

Psychiatric comorbidities

Psychiatric comorbidities in cerebral palsy

ScienciaScripts

Imprint

Any brand names and product names mentioned in this book are subject to trademark, brand or patent protection and are trademarks or registered trademarks of their respective holders. The use of brand names, product names, common names, trade names, product descriptions etc. even without a particular marking in this work is in no way to be construed to mean that such names may be regarded as unrestricted in respect of trademark and brand protection legislation and could thus be used by anyone.

Cover image: www.ingimage.com

This book is a translation from the original published under ISBN 978-613-9-73577-8.

Publisher:
Sciencia Scripts
is a trademark of
Dodo Books Indian Ocean Ltd. and OmniScriptum S.R.L publishing group

120 High Road, East Finchley, London, N2 9ED, United Kingdom
Str. Armeneasca 28/1, office 1, Chisinau MD-2012, Republic of Moldova, Europe
Printed at: see last page
ISBN: 978-620-7-87202-2

SUMMARY

CHAPTER 1

INTRODUCTION

Happy are those who go through life having a thousand reasons to live.
-Dom H and Ider Câmara

Cerebral palsy (CP), also known as "chronic non-progressive encephalopathy of childhood", is the result of a static lesion that occurred in the pre-, peri- or post-natal period, during the period of brain development, between birth and the second year of life. Any insult to the central nervous system (CNS) during this period of structural and functional maturation can subsequently cause CP (Bass, 1999).

Various clinical conditions can accompany CP, such as epilepsy and intellectual disability (ID). Psychiatric comorbidities such as Attention Deficit Hyperactivity Disorder (ADHD), Autism Spectrum Disorder (ASD), depression and anxiety, among others, seem to be more frequent in this population. However, few studies have actively investigated the presence of psychiatric disorders in children with CP.

The presence of psychiatric comorbidities worsens the functional and quality of life of these children. Early diagnosis and treatment should be part of the routine at rehabilitation centres. These centres focus on physical rehabilitation, and studies highlighting the need for a broader approach to people with CP are needed.

This work was born out of the perception of how much this reality is neglected in rehabilitation centres, how much the presence of comorbidity hinders rehabilitation, including motor rehabilitation, and how much its recognition and treatment have a positive impact on the lives of children and their families.

1.1. CEREBRAL PALSY

In 1860, William Little described for the first time a disorder with spasticity in the lower limbs and, to a lesser extent, in the upper limbs, which affected some children in the first years of life. The children had difficulty holding objects, crawling and walking and, over time, there was no improvement or worsening of the clinical picture. This condition, which became known as "Little's disease", is now recognised as spastic diplegia, one of the clinical forms of cerebral palsy (Diament, 1996).

Cerebral palsy has been described as a group of developmental disorders of movement and posture, attributed to a non-progressive disorder that occurs in the brain during foetal development or early childhood. The motor alterations observed in CP are often associated with sensory alterations, cognitive disorders, communication, perception, behaviour, as well as epilepsy (Bax *et al.,* 2005; Bjorgaas, Elgen, Boe, & Hysing, 2013; Rosenbaum *et al.,* 2007).

It is a predominantly sensorimotor dysfunction, involving disturbances in muscle tone, posture and voluntary movement. These disorders are characterised by a lack of control over movements, adaptive changes in muscle length and, in some cases, even bone deformities (Koman, Smith, & Shilt, 2004).

This disorder occurs during the period when children develop at an accelerated pace, i.e. in the first few years of life, and can compromise the process of acquiring skills. This impairment can interfere with function, hindering the performance of activities often carried out by children with normal development and increasing the risk of mental health problems (Parkes *et al.,* 2008).

Because of this definition and the predominance of motor symptoms in patients with CP, their treatment is practically aimed at motor improvement and is based on rehabilitation based on motor classification.

The prevalence of CP in developing countries is not well established, but it is estimated to be around 1.5 to 3.5 cases per 1,000 live births (Foster, Rai, Weller, Dixon, & Weller, 2010; Koman *et al.,* 2004; Lagault, Shevell, & Dagenais, 2011; Parkes & McCusker, 2008; Tilton & Delgado, 2011)

Although there are no population-based studies on the prevalence of CP in Brazil, it is known to be more common in poor or developing countries.

Physiologically, cerebral palsy can be divided into a spastic type, the most common (80 per cent), which affects the corticospinal (pyramidal) tract, and an extrapyramidal type, which affects the other regions of the developing brain, such as the basal nuclei and cerebellum. The extrapyramidal types of cerebral palsy include choreoathetoid, ataxic and hypotonic (Agarwal & Verma, 2012). Table 1 shows the differentiation of the clinical types of CP.

Table 1 - Differentiation of the clinical types of CP. Adapted from (Agarwal & Verma, 2012).

Clinical type	Features
Spastic	Increased muscle tone; joint contractures are common.
Choreoathetoid	Dyskinetic condition; involuntary movement;

	dystonia.
Ataxic	Movement coordination disorder; usually ambulatory; normal head segment control.
Hypotonic	Muscle hypotonia with normal tendon reflexes.
Mixed	More than one type in combination.

The Gross Motor Function Classification System (GMFCS) for cerebral palsy is based on voluntarily initiated movement, with an emphasis on motor acquisitions, transfers and mobility. This system is defined in five levels. When defining a five-level classification system, the main criterion is that the distinctions between the levels should be significant in daily life (Silva, Pfeifer, & Funayama, 2013).

The focus of the GMFCS is on determining which level best represents the child or young person's abilities and limitations in gross motor function. The emphasis should be on habitual performance in home, school and community settings (i.e. what they do - ability), rather than what they are known not to be able to do.

The distinctions are based on functional limitations, the need for manual mobility devices (such as walkers, crutches or canes) or mobility on wheels, and to a lesser extent, the quality of movement. The distinctions between Levels I and II are not as clear-cut as those between the other levels, particularly for children under two years of age (Palisano *etal.*, 1997). Table 2 shows the gross motor classification according to the GMFCS, and Table 3 shows the differentiation between the GMFCS levels.

Table 2 - Aerial characteristics of the GMFCS classification. Source: Silva *et al.* (2013).

GENERAL CHARACTERISTICS FOR EACH LEVEL	
Level 1	He walks without limitations.
Level II	He walks with limitations.
Level III	He walks using a manual mobility device.
Level IV	Limited self-mobility; can use motorised mobility.
Level V	Transported in a manual wheelchair.

Table 3 - Difference between levels in the GMFCS classification. Source: Silva *et al.* (2013).

DISTINCTIONS BETWEEN LEVELS	
Levels I-II	At level II, when compared to level 1 children, there are limitations to walking long distances and balancing; they may need a manual mobility device; they may use
	a wheeled device when walking long distances; require the use of handrails to go up and down stairs; and are unable to run and jump.

II-III levels	At level II, they are able to walk without a manual mobility device after the age of four. At level III, a manual mobility device is required for walking indoors and the use of wheeled mobility outside the home.
Levels III-IV	At level III, they sit on their own or require at most limited external support to sit; they are more independent in transferring to a standing posture and walk with a manual mobility device. At level IV, they sit, but self-movement is limited. At level IV, transport is more likely to be in a manual or motorised wheelchair.
Levels IV-V	At level V, there are severe limitations in head and trunk control and require extensive assistive technology and physical help. Self-movement is only achieved if the child/young person can learn how to operate a motorised wheelchair.

Mancini *et al.* (2002), comparing performance in functional self-care activities using the PEDI *(Paediatric Evaluation of Disability Inventory)* scale in children with normal development and children with cerebral palsy, found that the development of functional activities is influenced by CP. Although the sequence of skill acquisition is similar to that of children with normal development, the degree of difficulty of functional activities was much greater in the group with CP. This suggests that the brain that develops under the influence of injury and motor sequelae has different experiences and develops based on these experiences. Intervention must therefore take this characteristic into account.

Improvements in health care technology in recent years have significantly increased the number of children with CP who survive to adulthood. Children with mild to moderate CP have the same life expectancy as children without any chronic conditions. While in the past most attention was paid to the general survival care of these patients, today the emphasis is on their "life experience", i.e. their psychosocial adjustment and quality of life (Parkes & McCusker, 2008). In this context, thinking about the mental health of these patients is fundamental for a good quality of life, functionality, social and professional inclusion.

Current treatment models for CP focus on improving spasticity, controlling altered movements and deformities, and reducing the patient's physical discomfort. These treatment models focus solely on motor alterations. Determining how much these children and adolescents are at risk of psychiatric disorders has important implications for the treatment plan. Few studies have focused on intervention and prevention of psychiatric problems or on programmes that promote the mental health of this population (Bjorgaas *etal.,* 2013; Koman *etal.,* 2004; Parkes & McCusker, 2008).

1.2. PSYCHIATRIC COMORBIDITIES

CP has traditionally been seen as a motor control disorder. Thus, the focus of treatment has mainly been on aspects of its physical impairment. Treatable psychiatric syndromes in this population have been a neglected area of study. To date, few systematic studies of psychiatric comorbidities in children and adolescents with cerebral palsy have been conducted. This is worrying because children with CP apparently have a higher rate of psychiatric disorders than is expected for the rest of the population (Foster *et al,* 2010). Table 4 summarises the main studies related to psychiatric comorbidities in cerebral palsy.

Table 4 - Studies on psychiatric comorbidities in cerebral palsy.

Study / Year	Sample	Design	Conclusion
Goodman & Graham (1996)	428 children	Screening questionnaires	61% psychiatric comorbidities (3% ASD; 25% emotional problems; 13% ADHD)
Parkes *et al.* (2008)	818 children	*Strengths and Difficulties Questionnaire* (SDQ)	42% psychiatric comorbidities (29% emotional problems; 31% ADHD)
Foster et *al.* (2010)	1 teenager	Case report	Mood disorder
Brossard-Racine *et al.* (2012)	76 children	*Strengths and Difficulties Questionnaire* (SDQ) / Vineland Social Development Scale	39.4% behavioural problems; 55.3 per cent had difficulties with relationships with peers.
Bjorgaas, Hysing, & Elgen (2012)	67 children	Kiddie-Sads	57% with psychiatric comorbidities (16% anxiety; 15% ADHD; 37.3% LD)
Bjorgaas *et al.* (2013)	47 children	*Strengths and Difficulties Questionnaire* (SDQ)	57% with psychiatric comorbidities (51.1% ADHD; 8.5% ODD and 10.6% emotional problems)
Levy-Zaks, Pollak, & Ben-Pazi (2014)	18 children	*Child Behavior Checklist* (CBCL), *Disruptive Behavior Disorder Rating Scale* (DBDRS), *Pediatric Quality of Life Inventory* (PEDSQL)	13% internalising problems; 4% externalising

Despite the data available on the prevalence and severity of some comorbidities associated with CP (e.g. intellectual disability, sensory impairments and epilepsy), relatively little is known about the prevalence and severity of behavioural and emotional problems and their impact on the child and family (Parkes *et al.,* 2008).

In a classic study from 1968, Graham and Rutter, studying around 12,000 children on the Isle of Wight, observed a high rate of psychiatric disorders, five times higher than that of the general population, in individuals with epilepsy, cerebral palsy and other CNS pathologies; however, in this study, epilepsy was the significant factor for the presence of psychiatric disorders.

A higher prevalence of psychiatric problems is found in patients with CP when compared to control groups. The main problems encountered are difficulties in dealing with their peers, hyperactivity and emotional problems (Bjorgaas *etaL,* 2013; Parkes & McCusker, 2008).

The physical and mental health of the main carers of a child with a disability, most of whom are mothers, is inextricably linked to and strongly influenced by the child's behaviour and the care demanded of them (Raina *et al,* 2005).

Bostrõm, Broberg and Hwang (2010), studying the perception and impact of disability on fathers and mothers of children with various disabilities, observed in their subgroup analysis that children with Down's syndrome and cerebral palsy were described as having the least negative impact on their parents, while children with autism and intellectual disabilities were reported as having the greatest negative impact on their parents. Thus, diagnosing any psychiatric comorbidity, even ID in patients with CP, improves the family's approach and orientation regarding the possibilities and limitations of this individual.

The impact of disability on the family depends on various factors, but Boulet, Boyle and Schieve (2009), in a review of the impact of developmental disorders, found that cerebral palsy, autism, intellectual disability, blindness and deafness were the situations with the greatest functional impact on the child's life and care, and the situations that most led to the use of health services. This is important not only for family and community life, but also for public health, highlighting the need for public policies that take greater account of this group of patients.

Other authors, evaluating the positive impact of children with LD on their families, have shown that this was greater the fewer the behavioural problems. Managing children and adolescents with behavioural changes seems to be the biggest stress factor for families and schools (Blacher & Baker, 2007).

A study on quality of life in children with cerebral palsy, based on parental perception, found that it was lower the more severe the motor level (Vargus-Adams, 2005). The author also observed that behavioural changes were not detrimental to quality of life, however behaviour improved with the greater severity of CP, reflecting a difficulty in determining behavioural problems in children with global or severe deficits. The behavioural problems addressed in the scale used in the study include: arguing, lying and stealing, which, for children who cannot make conscious choices or act on these choices, may not occur. Thus, children with severe cerebral palsy may have been reported as behaving better, mainly because they did not have the ability to display bad behaviour. This phenomenon may explain the slight upward slope of the regression line for the behaviour domain found by the author.

Bjorgaas *et al.* (2013), evaluating *screening* scales for psychiatric disorders in children with CP, found that the SDQ *(Strengths and Difficulties Questionnaire) scale* was sensitive for this population, but was unable to predict certain disorders, especially ADHD.

Goodman and Graham (1996), studying children with hemiplegia, observed a rate of psychiatric disorders affecting 61% of the individuals assessed individually and 54% and 42% from parent and teacher questionnaires, respectively. Few of the children affected had been in contact with childhood mental health services. The strongest predictor of psychiatric problems was the intelligence quotient (QI), which was highly correlated with the neurological severity index. Age, gender and laterality of the injury had little or no power to predict the occurrence of psychiatric disorders.

Goodman (1998) reported that symptoms of "agitation" and "inattention" in pre-school children with hemiplegia were strong predictors of psychiatric problems in the six to 10 year-old age group. Interestingly, the author also found that adverse family conditions had little impact on the onset or remission of difficulties in children with hemiplegia, leading him to conclude that family factors are likely to be the consequence of psychiatric problems in children, rather than the cause.Early symptoms of inattention in preschool children with CP appear to be an important predictor of psychological problems at older ages. Early intervention in these symptoms may be the key to reducing anxiety and family stress and promoting better psychological adjustment in these children (Parkes & McCusker, 2008).

1.2.1. Anxiety and Depression

The first description of anxiety as a dysfunction of mental activity dates back to the early 19th century. In 1813, Augustin-Jacob Landré-Beuvais described anxiety as a syndrome composed of emotional aspects and physiological reactions. In 1844, Jean Baptiste Félix Descurate linked anxiety to illness in his book *The Medicine of the Passions.* In 1850, Otto Domrich first described what is now known as panic disorder. In 1871, Jacob Mendez da Costa reported new cases of panic, giving it the name "irritable heart syndrome". In 1880, Karl Westphal described the symptoms present in specific phobias and obsessive-compulsive disorder. In the paediatric population, the first clinical case reports of children with anxiety symptoms date back to the beginning of the 20th century (Vianna, Campos & Landeira-Fernandez, 2009).

Epidemiological studies in American populations have indicated that AD in children and adolescents has an estimated prevalence of 8% to 12% (Costello *et al*, 1988; Spence, 1998). In Brazil, a population study found prevalence rates of 4.6% in children and 5.8% among adolescents (Fleitlich-Bilyk & Goodman, 2004).

Anxiety is a very common clinical condition, possibly the most common psychopathology in childhood and adolescence, and its presence can have a negative impact on the child's life, requiring early diagnosis and treatment (Cartwright-Hatton, McNicol, & Doubleday, 2006; Martini, 1995). On the other hand, until the beginning of the 20th century, depression was considered very rare or non-existent in children. In recent years, studies have indicated a prevalence of 2% in the school population. Comorbidity between depression and anxiety is also commonly observed in this age group (Birmaher et *al.,* 2007; Brand-Gothelf, Yoeli-Bligh, Gilboa-Schechtman, Benaroya-Milshtein, & Apter, 2014).

Anxiety disorders include disorders that share characteristics of excessive fear and anxiety and related behavioural disturbances. They differ from adaptive fear and anxiety in that they are excessive or persist beyond periods appropriate to the level of development. These disorders are divided into: Separation Anxiety Disorder, Selective Mutism, Specific Phobia, Social Anxiety Disorder (Social Phobia), Panic Disorder, Agoraphobia and Generalised Anxiety Disorder (DSM - 5, 2013).

Depressive disorders include disruptive mood dysregulation disorder, major depressive disorder, persistent depressive disorder (dysthymia), premenstrual dysphoric disorder and depressive disorder not otherwise specified. Characteristic of these disorders is the presence of sad, empty or irritable mood, accompanied by somatic and cognitive changes that significantly affect the individual's ability to function (DSM - 5, 2013).

Few studies are found in the literature correlating internalising disorders and cerebral palsy. Levy-Zaks, Pollak and Ben-Pazi (2014), studying 18 children with CP, found a 13% rate of patients with internalising problems. In this study, no correlation was observed with the motor level of CP.

There are several difficulties with this diagnosis in the paediatric population, especially with CP. Parents of adolescents with CP do not report a high frequency of emotional problems, such as depression and anxiety. This situation is also observed with adolescents in general. Therefore, whenever possible, this investigation should be carried out with the adolescent themselves (Blackman & Conaway, 2014).

Pain is also a common experience for children and adolescents with cerebral palsy. Yamaguchi, Perry and Hines (2014) observed that the intensity of pain and the anxiety aroused by it have a strong association with behavioural and emotional problems in these patients and postulate that the healthcare team should consider how pain affects the emotional development of these children, taking this aspect into account in rehabilitation programmes. Actively researching pain and its consequences, especially in individuals with greater communication difficulties, is part of a broader and more appropriate approach to this condition.

The evidence base for psychological disorders in children with chronic illnesses and disabilities in general has sometimes been contradictory. While some studies have documented the presence of psychological alterations, others have found little or no results. Determining whether these children are at greater risk for psychiatric disorders has important implications for planning health resources and services (Parkes & McCusker, 2008).

Brain damage, cognitive impairment, social stigma and learning difficulties increase the likelihood of psychiatric disorders. It is postulated that brain damage itself may be a vulnerability factor for the occurrence of psychiatric disorders. However, it is unclear whether brain dysfunction leads directly to behavioural disorders or causes an increase in the child's vulnerability to environmental stress, secondarily causing these alterations (Foster *etal.,* 2010).

1.2.2. Attention Deficit Hyperactivity Disorder

The story of ADHD usually begins with Heinrich Hoffman's great book *Struwwelpeter* - which translates as "Sloppy Peter". In this book, although the aim was not to describe a psychopathology, the author already described the symptoms of the disorder. At the beginning of the 20th century, the idea of Minimal Brain Dysfunction gained strength to explain excessively restless children.

Later, in the 1970s, a powerful step came from Dykman *et al.* (1971) in formulating minimal brain dysfunction as an attention disorder, emphasising poor performance and increased reaction time. This was the beginning of the development of the key idea of Attention Deficit Disorder, which came with DSM-III, the third edition of the *Diagnostic and Statistical Manual of* the American Psychiatric Association (American Psychiatric Association, 1980). This was of great importance in the development of child psychiatry because it replaced the etiological formulations of the past (which were unreliable due to the difficulty of attributing causes to cases) with a simple description of observable behaviours (Taylor, 2011).

Attention Deficit Hyperactivity Disorder is an early onset neurobehavioural condition that persists into adolescence and adulthood, with a high prevalence, clinically heterogeneous, with a significant cost to society, both in economic terms and in terms of academic prognosis and family stress. It has a neurobiological basis and affects both sexes. The deficit includes academic and social dysfunction, with a high risk in adolescence of school failure, low self-esteem, relationship difficulties, parental conflicts, delinquency and substance abuse. It is characterised by symptoms of inattention, hyperactivity and impulsivity throughout life (Biederman, 2005). It is a disorder with a high prevalence, estimated to affect 5-10% of children worldwide (Faraone, Sergeant, Gillberg, & Biederman, 2003).

Table 5 shows the diagnostic criteria for ADHD according to the DSM-5.

Table 5 - Diagnostic criteria for ADHD.

Diagnostic Criteria for Attention Deficit/Hyperactivity Disorder
A. A persistent pattern of inattention and/or hyperactivity-impulsivity that interferes with functioning and development, as characterised by (1) and/or (2):
1. **Inattention:** Six (or more) of the following symptoms persist for at least six months to a degree that is inconsistent with developmental level and have a direct negative impact on social and academic/professional activities:
a. They often don't pay attention to details or make careless mistakes in schoolwork, at work or during other activities (for example, they neglect or miss details, their work is inaccurate).
b. They often have difficulty keeping their attention on tasks or leisure activities (for example, difficulty staying focused during lessons, conversations or prolonged reading).
c. They often don't seem to listen when someone addresses them directly (for example, they seem to have their head turned away, even in the absence of any obvious distraction).
d. They often don't follow instructions through to the end and can't finish schoolwork, tasks or duties in the workplace (for example, they start tasks but quickly lose focus and easily lose their way).
e. They often have difficulty organising tasks and activities (e.g. difficulty managing sequential tasks; difficulty keeping materials and personal belongings in order; disorganised and sloppy work; poor time management; difficulty meeting deadlines).
f. Often avoids, dislikes or is reluctant to get involved in tasks that require prolonged mental effort (for example, schoolwork or homework; for older teenagers and adults, preparing reports,
filling in forms, proofreading long papers).

g- They often lose things they need for tasks or activities (e.g. school materials, pencils, books, instruments, desks, keys, documents, glasses, mobile phones).

h. They are often easily distracted by external stimuli (for older adolescents and adults, this can include unrelated thoughts).

i. It's often forgotten when it comes to everyday activities (for example, doing chores, obligations; for older teenagers and adults, returning calls, paying bills, keeping appointments).

2. **Hyperactivity and impulsivity:** Six (or more) of the following symptoms persist for at least six months to a degree that is inconsistent with developmental level and have a direct negative impact on social and academic/professional activities:

a. They often fidget or tap their hands or feet or squirm in their chair.

b. Frequently gets up from his chair in situations where he is expected to remain seated (for example, gets out of his seat in class, in the office or other workplace or in other situations that require him to remain in one place).

c. Often runs or climbs on things in situations where this is inappropriate.

d. They are often unable to play or engage in leisure activities calmly.

e. They often "won't stop", acting as if they have "the engine running" (for example, they can't or feel uncomfortable sitting still for a long time, such as in restaurants, meetings; others may see them as restless or difficult to keep up with).

f. He often talks too much.

g- They often let an answer slip before the question has been completed (for example, they finish other people's sentences, they can't wait for their turn to speak).

h. They often have difficulty waiting their turn (for example, waiting in a queue).

i. Often interrupts or intrudes (e.g. butts into conversations, games or activities; may start using other people's things without asking or receiving permission; for teenagers and adults, may intrude on or take control of what others are doing).

B. Several symptoms of inattention or hyperactivity-impulsivity were present before the age of 12.

C. Several symptoms of inattention or hyperactivity-impulsivity are present in two or more environments (for example, at home, at school, at work, with friends or relatives; in other activities).

D. There is clear evidence that the symptoms interfere with or reduce the quality of social, academic or professional functioning.

E. The symptoms do not occur exclusively during the course of schizophrenia or another psychotic disorder and are not better explained by another mental disorder (e.g. mood disorder, anxiety disorder, dissociative disorder, personality disorder, substance intoxication or withdrawal).

Bjorgaas, Hysing and Elgen (2012) found more than 50 per cent of psychiatric comorbidities in 56 children with CP, and of these, the main comorbidity was ADHD, followed by anxiety. Epilepsy was not a significant factor in the prevalence of psychiatric disorders. The authors observed no correlation with the level or type of CP. However, a higher incidence of psychiatric disorders was found in those patients with greater communication problems. Autism spectrum disorders were not investigated in this study.

The complexity of CP poses a challenge for the diagnosis of ADHD, and differentiating between other causes of inattention, such as epileptic changes, intellectual disability and chronic pain, as well as communication difficulties, and sleep disorders, is the great challenge of this condition (Newman, 0'Regan, & Hensey, 2006).

Children and adolescents with CP should be regularly screened by healthcare providers actively looking for the occurrence of mental health problems, with a focus on emotional, behavioural, academic and social problems. Care should be taken in the assessment and intervention of children with CP to ensure that psychological problems are not overlooked and potentially preventable risk factors are identified and treated early and effectively, thus improving the quality of life of children and their families (Foster *et al.*, 2010).

1.2.3. Autism Spectrum Disorders

The word "autism" comes from the Greek *autos,* which means "turning in on oneself". The first person to use it was the Austrian psychiatrist Eugen Bleuler, in 1911, to refer to one of the criteria adopted at the time for making a diagnosis of schizophrenia. These criteria became known as "Bleuler's four A's": hallucinations, disorganised affect, incongruence and autism.

The word "autism" referred to the schizophrenic's tendency to "wall themselves off", becoming oblivious to the social world - closing themselves off from it.

In 1943, the Austrian child psychiatrist Leo Kanner studied 11 patients with a diagnosis of schizophrenia more closely and observed autism as the most striking feature. He then used the term *"Autistic Disturbance of Affective Contact"* to describe the condition, which was characterised by extreme isolation, obsessive behaviour and stereotyping.

In 1944, Austrian paediatrician Hans Asperger proposed in his study the definition of a disorder that he called *"Autistic Psychopathy",* manifested by a severe disorder in social interaction, pedantic use of speech, motor maladjustment and incidence only in males. The author used the description of some clinical cases, characterising the family history, physical and behavioural aspects, performance in intelligence tests, as well as emphasising the concern with the educational approach of these individuals (APUD Assumpção Jr, 2000).

Autism and related autism spectrum conditions are chronic conditions whose behavioural manifestations include qualitative deficits in social interaction and communication, repetitive and stereotyped patterns of behaviour and a restricted repertoire of interests and activities (DSM - 5, 2013).

The epidemiology of ASD is approximately two to five cases per 1,000 children, predominantly in males. This prevalence has been increasing in recent decades, especially due to earlier diagnosis, associated with better and broader definition of diagnostic criteria (Lenoir *etal.,* 2009; Rapin, 2002). Fombone (2009) speaks of a 1% prevalence, while Zablotski, Black, Maenner, Schieve, and Blumberg (2015) speak of 2.4%.

Today, ASD is defined as a behavioural syndrome with defined organic etiologies. According to Gillberg (1990), autism is an organic dysfunction and the new way of looking at autism is biological.

Research supports the view of autism spectrum disorders as an expression of atypical brain development, which results in more or less widespread dysfunctions (and not necessarily with a specific aetiology) that are complex and widely distributed in the neural network. The diagnosis of ASD is based mainly on the patient's clinical picture, and there is still no single biological marker to characterise it (Costa & Nunesmaia, 1998).

The criteria currently used to diagnose autism are described in the American Psychiatric Association's *Diagnostic and Statistical Manual,* DSM-5, and according to this the behavioural manifestations that define autism include qualitative deficits in social interaction and communication, repetitive and stereotyped patterns of behaviour and a restricted repertoire of interests and activities.

Table 6 shows the diagnostic criteria for ASD according to the DSM-5.

Table 6 - Diagnostic criteria for Autism Spectrum Disorder.

A. Persistent deficits in social communication and social interaction in multiple contexts, as manifested by the following, currently or by previous history:

1. Deficit in socio-emotional reciprocity, ranging, for example, from abnormal social approach and difficulty establishing normal conversation to reduced sharing of interests, emotions or affection, to difficulty initiating or responding to social interactions.

2. Deficits in non-verbal communicative behaviours used for social integration, ranging, for example, from poorly integrated verbal and non-verbal communication to abnormalities in eye contact and body language or deficits in the understanding and use of gestures, the total absence of facial expressions and non-verbal communication.

3. Deficits in developing, maintaining and understanding relationships, ranging, for example, from difficulty in adjusting behaviour to suit different social contexts, to difficulty in sharing imaginative play or making friends, to a lack of interest in peers.

Severity is based on impairments in social communication and restricted, repetitive behaviour patterns.

B. Restricted and repetitive patterns of behaviour, interests or activities, as manifested by at least two of the following, currently or from previous history:

1. Stereotyped or repetitive motor movements, use of objects or speech (e.g. simple motor stereotypies, lining up toys or spinning objects, echolalia, idiosyncratic phrases).

2. Insistence on the same things, inflexible adherence to routines or ritualised patterns of verbal or non-verbal behaviour (for example, extreme distress at small changes, difficulties with transitions, rigid patterns of thought, greeting rituals, the need to take the same route or eat the same food every day).

3. Fixed and highly restricted interests that are abnormal in intensity or focus (e.g. for example, strong attachment to, or preoccupation with, unusual objects, excessively circumscribed or perseverative interests).

4. Hyper- or hyporeactivity to sensory stimuli or unusual interest in sensory aspects of the environment (e.g. apparent indifference to pain/temperature, contrary reaction to specific sounds or textures, excessive smelling or touching of objects, visual fascination with lights or movement).

Severity is based on impairments in social communication and restricted or repetitive patterns of behaviour.

C. Symptoms must be present early in the developmental period (but may not become fully manifest until social demands exceed limited capacities) or may be masked by strategies learnt later in life.

D. The symptoms cause clinically significant impairment in the individual's present social, occupational or other important areas of life.

E. These disorders are no longer best explained by intellectual disability (intellectual development disorder) or global developmental delay.

Table 7 shows the severity specifiers that can be used to describe the current symptomatology, recognising that severity can vary with the context or fluctuate over time, according to the DSM-5.

Table 7 - Severity levels for Autism Spectrum Disorder.

Severity Level	Social Communication	Restricted and repetitive behaviour
Level 3 "Requiring very substantial support"	Severe deficits in verbal and non-verbal social communication skills cause severe impairments in functioning, great limitations in initiating social interactions and minimal response to social overtures from others. For example, a person with unintelligible speech of a few words who rarely initiates interactions and, when they do, has unusual approaches	Inflexibility of behaviour, extreme difficulty in coping with change or other restricted / repetitive behaviours interfere markedly with functioning in all spheres. Great suffering /
	only to satisfy needs and reacts only to very direct social approaches.	difficulty changing focus or actions.
Level 2	Severe deficits in verbal and non-verbal	Inflexibility of behaviour,

"Requiring substantial support"	social communication skills; apparent social impairments even in the presence of support; limitation in initiating social interactions and reduced or abnormal response to social overtures from others. For example, a person who speaks in simple sentences, whose interaction is limited to narrow special interests and who displays markedly awkward non-verbal communication.	difficulty coping with change or other restricted/repetitive behaviours appear frequently enough to be obvious to the casual observer and interfere with functioning in a variety of contexts. Suffering and/or difficulty changing focus or actions.
Level 1 "Demanding support"	In the absence of support, deficits in social communication cause notable damage. Difficulty initiating social interactions and clear examples of atypical or unsuccessful responses to social overtures from others. May appear to show reduced interest in social interactions. For example, a person who is able to speak in full sentences and engage in communication, but who fails to converse with others and whose attempts to make friends are awkward and often unsuccessful.	Inflexibility of behaviour causes significant interference in functioning in one or more contexts. Difficulty switching activities. Problems with organisation and planning are obstacles to independence.

The prevalence of ASD in patients with cerebral palsy is around 15%. Kilincaslan and Mukaddes (2009), studying 126 children with CP, observed a rate of 11% and 4% of patients with autism and invasive developmental disorder, respectively, using the DSM - IV - TR criteria. The type of CP (tetraespastic and hemiplegic), the presence of epilepsy and the intellectual level were the relevant differences between the groups.

Goodman and Graham (1996) found a 3% prevalence of ASD in patients with hemiplegia. In this study, there were no differences in gender, age or laterality of the lesion.

Kirby *et al.* (2011), in a multicentre study in the United States, found a prevalence of 8% of ASD in children with CP. It varied from 3-12% depending on the area and they also observed that the frequency of ASD decreased as the severity of the motor condition increased, which they considered to be the acquisition of gait.

The association between epilepsy and CP is very evident and the latter with autism is also proving to be prevalent. Spencer and Schneider (2009), in a literature review, found some characteristics associated with a higher incidence of epilepsy in autistic people, such as low IQ, associations with neurogenetic diseases, developmental regression and gender (female).

Binnie and Marston (1992) suggested that epileptiform paroxysms without clinical seizures could lead to cognitive disorders. Studying patients with roland epilepsy, the authors observed what they called transient cognitive loss. However, it is not possible to say that all patients with subclinical epileptiform discharges have this cognitive loss and that this negatively affects their psychosocial functioning. But considering this hypothesis and the higher prevalence of epilepsy in patients with CP, this may be a factor in the higher occurrence of LD and other cognitive alterations observed in this group.

Gabis, Pomeroy and Andriola (2005) retrospectively studied 56 patients with autism, TID and Asperger's Syndrome and observed a significantly higher incidence of epilepsy in autistic patients, supporting the hypothesis that these phenomena are comorbid and are a common brain abnormality. This hypothesis corroborates the prerogative that brains with developmental disorders or that develop concomitantly with a pathological or lesion process are at increased risk of other clinical situations.

As for gender, girls with autism have a higher incidence of epilepsy than boys, which is probably due to the greater association of intellectual disability associated with autism in this population. Although intellectual disability increases the

 risk of epilepsy, it seems that autism alone is associated with higher rates of epilepsy (Gadia, Tuchman, & Rotta, 2004; Spence & Schneider, 2009; Tuchman, Rapin, & Shinnar, 1991).

 Desai *et al.* (2012), studying the impact of autism on family members in Goa, India, proposed that the parents' experience involves four temporal phases: Phase one - a period of celebration; phase two - the perception of unexpected behaviour; phase three - the parents' observation in public situations; and phase four - where the parents recognise the persistence of behavioural changes.In phases one and two, the word autism is not yet present and the parents still understand it as a specific delay, for example in speech. In stage three, the persistence of difficulties indicates autism, but the long-term prognosis is only understood in stage four. In this sense, parents of individuals with CP need more support to receive a second diagnosis.

1.2.4. Intellectual Disability

Intellectual disability is a disorder beginning in the period of neuropsychomotor development characterised by deficits in general mental abilities, such as reasoning, problem solving, planning, abstract thinking, judgement, academic learning and learning from experience. The deficits result in functional impairment, both intellectual and adaptive, in the conceptual, social and practical domains. Adaptation to the environment is always affected in the current part of the diagnostic criteria (DSM - 5, 2013). For LD, the score for levels of intellectual development should be determined on the basis of all available information, including clinical signs, adaptive behaviour in the cultural environment, individual results and psychometric tests. Its presence has a huge social effect, not only affecting the people who have the diagnosis, but also their families and society as a whole. Its prevalence is estimated at 1% to 3% in developed countries (Katz & Lazcano-Ponce, 2008).

For the DSM-5 *(Diagnostic and Statistical Manual of Mental Disorders* 5ª Ed.), the diagnosis of intellectual disability is based on three important criteria: Criterion A: Intelligence Quotient below 70; Criterion B: Significant limitations in adaptive functioning in at least two of the following skill areas: communication, self-care, domestic life, social/interpersonal skills, use of community resources, self-reliance, academic skills, work, leisure, health and safety; Criterion C: Occurring before the age of 18.

The association of LD with cerebral palsy varies between 25% and 50% in various studies (Andersen *et al.,* 2008; Himmelmann, Beckung, Hagberg, & Uvebrant, 2006; Huang, Tseng, Chen, Shieh, & Lu, 2013; Koman et al., 2004; Singhi & Saini, 2013; Tan *et al.,* 2014). This association causes limitations especially in learning and is linked to the degree of brain involvement (Koman *et al.,* 2004).

In a Norwegian study, the authors observed the presence of DL in 31 per cent of the 85 children assessed, which was more frequent in tetra-spastic forms of CP (Andersen *et al.,* 2008). Himmelmann *et al.* (2006) found LD in 40 per cent of their sample. They also observed that the proportion of children with associated losses (SLD, visual and hearing impairment) increased significantly according to GMFCS level, with 79% of children at level I having no comorbidities, in contrast to 6% at level V.

Several factors determine the overall performance of children with CP. The severity of the motor impairment and intellectual disability, as well as contextual factors such as the educational assistant and educational performance. In addition, it is important to mention that the child's pro-social behaviour has a positive impact on the performance of cognitive/behavioural activities at school (Huang *et al.,* 2013).

When we look at the participation of adolescents in social activities, the severity of the motor condition and the intellectual disability are the factors that have the greatest impact on the frequency of this participation. Adolescents with a single mild disability participated in some social domains as frequently as adolescents in the general population (Michelsen *etal.,* 2014).

Intellectual disability is more characteristic for the development of social and adaptive participation than the GMFCS level. Developmental trajectories and the diagnosis of ID can improve support for individuals with CP and their families in setting realistic goals and optimising the choice of interventions at an early age (Tan *etal.,* 2014).

The results of studies related to the schooling of children and adolescents with CP can serve as a guide for health services to prioritise activities, plan assessment and appropriate intervention for children with CP who have limitations in activity performance at school (Huang *etal.,* 2013).

CHAPTER 2

BACKGROUND

God is in the coincidences.

-Nelson Rodrigues

Rehabilitation programmes for cerebral palsy patients focus on motor gains. There is no routine psychiatric assessment in most care centres, nor is there a specific focus on comorbidities.

The presence of psychiatric comorbidities worsens the functional and quality of life of these children, which is why their recognition and treatment should be part of the routine in rehabilitation centres. Early diagnosis is essential for more complete treatment.

Below are two illustrative cases that highlight the importance of this research.

Case 1: G.W.S., 3 years and 6 months old, diagnosed with spastic diparetic cerebral palsy, motor level III, undergoing unsuccessful gait training with a walker. The patient does not accept the use of a suropodalic positioning orthosis and does not co-operate with therapy. A PSC assessment was carried out, which was positive, with a subsequent ATA assessment, which scored 32 (ASD). Psychological and occupational therapy intervention was carried out, with desensitisation of the feet to use the orthosis and behavioural training alongside physiotherapy. The patient progressed well with the completion of gait training and use of the aids.

Case 2: G., 14 years old, diagnosed with spastic diparetic cerebral palsy, motor level III, undergoing gait training with a walker after surgery. The minor complained of migratory pain, irritability and no adherence to gait training. After a positive CSP, a clinical assessment was carried out with a final diagnosis of depression. Drug therapy was introduced in association with psychotherapy and after five weeks the patient was able to walk again without complaining of pain.

2.1 OBJECTIVES

2.1.1. GENERAL

To investigate the prevalence of psychiatric comorbidities in children and adolescents with cerebral palsy treated at a tertiary rehabilitation centre.

2.1.2. SPECIFIC

To study Autism Spectrum Disorders (ASD) and Attention Deficit Hyperactivity Disorder (ADHD) separately, comparing them with the type of CP, age, gender and the presence or absence of epilepsy.

Also compare the impact on functionality of patients with ASD/ADHD with patients with CP without other comorbidities, matched by age and motor level.

CHAPTER 3

EVERYTHING

Man is a small world.
-Arist ó teles

This is an observational, prospective, cross-sectional study. For the research project, 550 individuals diagnosed with cerebral palsy were studied and treated at a tertiary physical rehabilitation centre (Associação de Assistência à Criança Deficiente - AACD - Osasco Unit). All the patients had their motor condition classified according to the GMFCS.

The individuals were screened using the PSC scale for psychiatric symptoms *(Paediatric Symptom Checklist)* (Appendix A), validated in Brazil by Muzzolon, Cat and Santos (2013) and then, if they scored above the average cut-off, they were assessed by two examiners separately.

The psychiatric diagnosis was made according to the parameters of the DSM-5 and ICD-10, as well as the autistic traits scale - ATA (Assumpção Júnior *et al.,* 2008) for ASD (Appendix B) and the SNAP IV for ADHD (Appendix C).

The CGAS *(Children's Global Assessment Scale)* (Shaffer *et al.,* 1983) was used to check the adaptive impact and compare the sample of autism spectrum disorders with CP (Appendix D).

Intelligence was assessed using the WISC IV, WAIS III or Columbia, depending on age, by a neuropsychologist from the department. The Vineland Social Development Scale (Sparrow SS, Baila DA, & DV, 1984) was the instrument used to check adaptive behaviour (Appendix E).

3.1. INSTRUMENTS
- PSC - *Paediatric Symptom Checklist* is a screening tool for emotional and/or psychosocial problems in children and adolescents aged 6-16.

  years. It consists of a 35-item questionnaire administered to parents or carers, which reflects their impression of the child's behaviour and development. The cut-off point for positive risk is > 28 points (Muzzolon *et al.,* 2013).

- ATA - autistic traits scale: this is a scale made up of 23 sub-scales divided into different items. Each subscale is scored from 0 to 2, according to the number of positive items (0 points for no items, 1 point for 1 item and 2 points for two or more items); the overall score is calculated from the arithmetic sum of the points on the subscales, and a score of more than 23 points is suggestive of a diagnosis of ASD (Assumpção Júnior *et al.,* 2008).

- SNAP IV: this is a questionnaire in the public domain, a successor to SNAP-III and SNAP-IIIR, the latter two formulated from the third version of the DSM and its revision, respectively, all using a four-level severity scale. This scale was revised by Swanson, Nolan and Pelham in 1983 and validated in Brazil by Matos *et al.* (2006).

- Weschler Intelligence Scale for Children - 4ª Edition (WISC IV): applied by a neuropsychologist from the rehabilitation centre team. The Wechsler Intelligence Scale for Children is an individually applied clinical instrument designed to assess children's intellectual capacity and problem-solving processes. Age range: six years and zero months to 16 years and 11 months. It consists of 15 subtests, 10 of which are main and five supplementary, and has four indices, namely: Verbal Comprehension index, Perceptual Organisation index, Operational Memory index and Processing Speed index, as well as the Total IQ.
- Weschler Intelligence Scale for adults - WAIS III: applied by a neuropsychologist from the rehabilitation centre team. It is a test for the clinical assessment of the intellectual capacity of adults aged between 16 and 89.
- Columbia Mental Maturity Scale: non-verbal intelligence test administered by a neuropsychologist from the rehabilitation centre team. The aim of this test is to assess the intellectual capacity of children in general through non-verbal responses. The material used for the Columbia Mental Scale consists of cards with printed drawings. The drawings on the cards are geometric figures, people, animals, plants or objects common in children's experience. The aim is to find the figure that is different from the others, with the difference becoming more complex, involving problems of analogy and abstract relationships.
-CGAS - *Children's Global Assessment Scale:* this is a nine-item scale that measures the global functioning of children and adolescents. It scores the subject's most impaired level of general functioning for a specific period of time of one month, selecting the lowest level that describes their functioning on a hypothetical health-disease *continuum.* Current functioning is scored, regardless of treatment or

prognosis (Shaffer *et al.,* 1983).

-Vineland Adaptive Behaviour Scale : assesses the patient's functional level in four areas: communication, activities of daily living, socialisation and motor skills, measuring a development quotient (Sparrow SS *et al,* 1984).

3.2. PARTICIPANTS

3.2.1 Inclusion criteria

Patients with cerebral palsy aged between 1-17 years and 11 months whose parents or guardians have signed an informed consent form.

3.2.2 Exclusion Criteria

For patients in the comorbid ADHD group, those with moderate to severe LD were excluded;

Patients with neuromuscular or degenerative diseases;

Patients with other associated sensory impairments (visual or hearing).

3.3. ANALYSING THE DATA

The SPSS statistical package (version 18.0) for the Windows operating system was used to analyse the data. A statistically significant value was considered to be $p<0.05$. Descriptive analyses were used to verify the distribution of individuals according to demographic data, CP characteristics (i.e. type and motor level) and the presence of comorbidities (i.e. epilepsy, intellectual disability and Axis I psychiatric disorders). We used the chi-squared test to determine possible differences in the distribution of subjects between different categories (i.e. sex, type of CP and level of CP in patients with ASD, ADHD and controls; presence of psychiatric disorder and type of CP; relative risk of having epilepsy or intellectual disability in patients with ASD). Differences in CGAS scores between the ASD, ADHD and control groups were checked using the Kruskall-Wallis test.

3.4 ETHICAL ASPECTS

Informed Consent Form - Appendix F

As a condition for taking part in the study, the parents or guardians of each participant will sign a free and informed consent form, with clarifications about the research and information regarding risks and confidentiality. This form has been drawn up in accordance with CNS Resolution 466/2012, according to the Council of the European Union.

National Health Council (CNS). Available at:

<http://www.ip.usp.br/portal/index.php?option=com_content&view=article&id=312&Itemi

d=283&lang=en>.

The research was approved by the Research Ethics Committee through the Brazil Platform Opinion Number: 1.007.076 Reporting Date: 26/01/2015 (Appendix G).

CHAPTER 4

RESULTS

I realise that my work is a drop in the ocean,

But without him, the ocean would be smaller.

-Madre Teresa of Calcutta d

1. Description of the sample in terms of type of CP and motor level

550 individuals diagnosed with cerebral palsy were assessed, 316 (57.45%) males and 234 (42.54%) females, with a mean age of 8.99 years (± 4.96, ranging from one to 18 years) and a median age of 9.00 years (Q1-Q3: 5-13).

As for the classification of cerebral palsy, 490 patients (89.09%) had the spastic form, with 180 (32.73%) spastic diparetic, 204 (37.09%) spastic tetraparetic and 106 (19.27%) spastic hemiparetic (55 on the right and 51 on the left).

The choreoathetoid form was observed in 39 (7.09%) patients, in six (1.09%) the form was ataxic and 15 (2.73%) patients had a mixed form (spastic associated with choreoathetoid) (Figure 1).

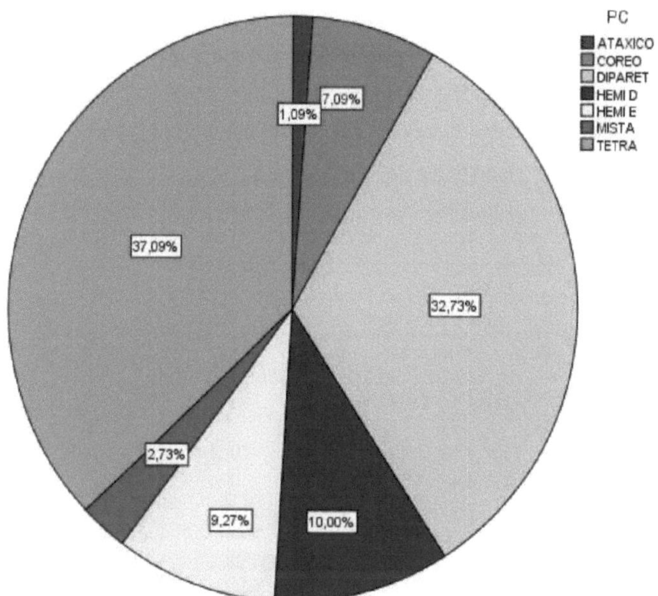

Figure 1- Classification of cerebral palsy.
Key: DIPARET: spastic diparetic; TETRA: spastic tetraparetic; HEMI: spastic hemiparetic; D: right; E: left; COREO: choreoathetoid.

When the association between motor level and cerebral palsy classification was checked, the following distribution was observed, as shown in Table 8.

Table 8 - Distribution of subjects according to the type of cerebral palsy and their motor level.

		LEVEL				
		1	II	III	IV	V
		N (%)	N (%)	N (%)	N (%)	N (%)
PC	ATXIC	3 (50%)	3 (50%)	0	0	0
	COREO	5(12,5%)	6(15%)	6(15%)	7(17,5%)	15(37,5%)
	Diparetic	57 (31,7%)	42 (23,3%)	42 (23,3%)	36 (20%)	3(1,7%)
	HEMI D	44 (80%)	6(10,9%)	3 (5,5%)	2 (3,6%)	0
	HEMI E	33 (64,7%)	12(23,5%)	4 (7,8%)	2 (3,9%)	0
	MIXED	1 (6,7%)	0	5 (33%)	3 (20%)	6 (40%)
	TETRA	0	0	17(8,3%)	83 (40,7%)	104(51%)

Key: Diparetic: spastic diparetic; TETRA: spastic tetraparetic; HEMI: spastic hemiparetic; D: right; E: left; COREO: choreoathetoid.

2 *Clinical form* and *level of severity of CP in patients with intellectual disabilities*

The most frequently observed psychiatric comorbidity was intellectual disability in 283 (44.55%) of the patients. Of these, 47 (16.6%) had mild ID, 121 (42.75%) had moderate ID and 115 (40.63%) had severe or profound ID.

When we selected only the subjects with intellectual disabilities (n=283), we found that 265 patients (93.6%) had the spastic form, 59 (20.8%) spastic diparetic, 181 (64%) spastic tetraparetic and 25 (8.8%) spastic hemiparetic (11 on the right and 14 on the left). The choreoathetoid form was observed in 10 (3.5%) patients, in two (0.7%) the form was ataxic and 6 (2.1%) patients had a mixed form (spastic associated with choreoathetoid).

The association between motor level and the classification of cerebral palsy in patients with intellectual disabilities is shown in Table 9, its correlation with the type of CP and motor level in Table 10 and the gender distribution in Table 11.

Table 9 - Distribution of subjects with intellectual disabilities according to the type of cerebral palsy and its level.

		LEVEL					Total
		1	II	III	IV	V	
PC	ATXIC	2(100%)	0	0	0	0	2
	COREO	1 (10%)	0	1 (10%)	3 (30%)	5 (50%)	10
	Diparetic	9 (15,3%)	11 (18,6%)	15 (25,4%)	21 (35,6%)	3(5,1%)	59
	HEMI D	3 (27,3%)	3 (27,3%)	3 (27,3%)	2(18,2%)	0	11
	HEMI E	5 (35,7%)	4 (28,6%)	3(21,4%)	2 (14,3%)	0	14
	MIXED	0	0	1 (16,7%)	0	5 (83,3%)	6
	TETRA	0	0	7 (3,9%)	72 (39,8%)	102 (56,4%)	181
Total		20	18	30	100	115	283

Key: Diparetic: spastic diparetic; TETRA: spastic tetraparetic; HEMI: spastic hemiparetic; D: right; E: left; COREO: choreoathetoid.

Table 10 - Distribution of patients with intellectual disabilities according to type of CP and motor level.

			LEVEL					Total
			1	II	III	IV	V	
PC	ATXIC	Count	2	0	0	0	0	2
		% within PC	100,0%	,0%	,0%	,0%	,0%	100,0%
	COREO	Count	1	0	1	3	5	10
		% within PC	10,0%	,0%	10,0%	30,0%	50,0%	100,0%
	DIPARET	Count	9	11	15	21	3	59
		% within PC	15,3%	18,6%	25,4%	35,6%	5,1%	100,0%
	HEMI D	Count	3	3	3	2	0	11
		% within PC	27,3%	27,3%	27,3%	18,2%	,0%	100,0%
	HEMI E	Count	5	4	3	2	0	14
		% within PC	35,7%	28,6%	21,4%	14,3%	,0%	100,0%
	Mixed	Count	0	0	1	0	5	6
		% within PC	,0%	,0%	16,7%	,0%	83,3%	100,0%
	TETRA	Count	0	0	7	72	102	181
		% within PC	,0%	,0%	3,9%	39,8%	56,4%	100,0%
Total		Count	20	18	30	100	115	283
		% within PC	7,1%	6,4%	10,6%	35,3%	40,6%	100,0%

Table 11 - Distribution of patients with CP according to the presence of intellectual disability and gender.

			Gender		Total
			M	F	
AXIS II - DI	Absent	Count	161	106	267
		%	60,3%	39,7%	100,0%
	DI	Count	155	128	283
		%	54,8%	45,2%	100,0%
Total		Count	316	234	550

| | | % | 57,5% | 42,5% | 100,0% |

Patients with and without intellectual disabilities had a similar gender distribution (x2=1.72; p=0.190).

3 Description of the sample in terms of the presence of epilepsy

Next, we investigated the presence of comorbidities in the patients. Epilepsy was observed in 238 (43.2%) patients (Figure 2).

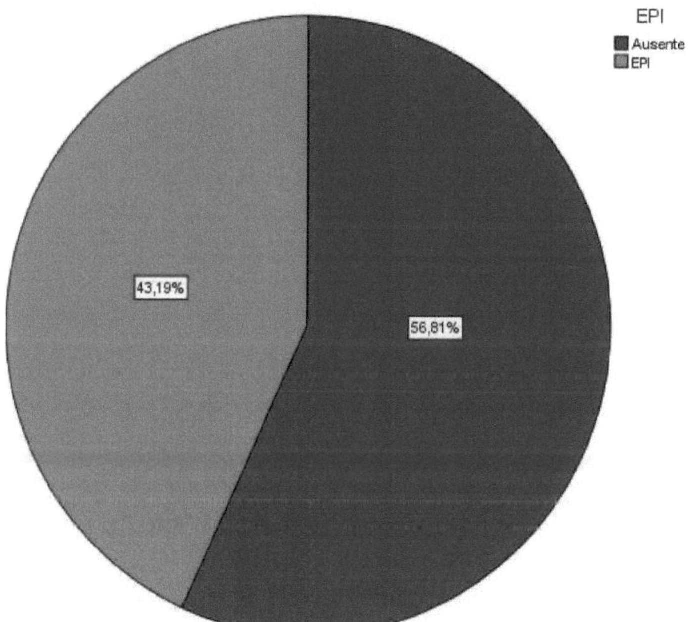

Figure 2 - Frequency of epilepsy in patients with cerebral palsy.
Caption: EPI: epilepsy.

4. Description of the sample in terms of the presence of psychiatric disorders

With regard to the presence of psychiatric comorbidities, we found that 337 (61.3 per cent) met the criteria for an Axis I or II psychiatric disorder (Figure 3).

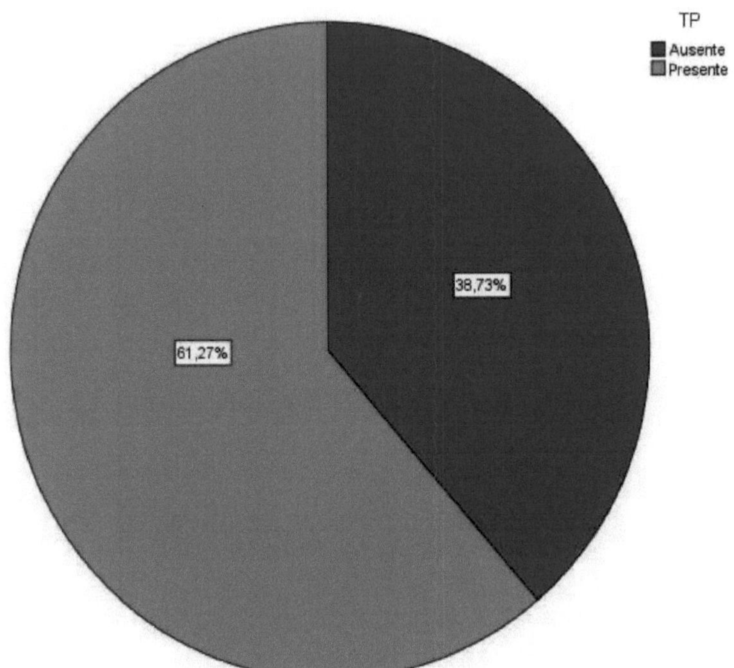

Figure 3 - Frequency of psychiatric disorders.
Caption: PT: psychiatric disorder.

In order to explore in more detail the presence of psychiatric comorbidities in patients with CP, we separated the sample into four categories: (i) patients with no psychiatric comorbidity (Axis I and II); (ii) patients with Axis I psychiatric disorders; (iii) patients with intellectual disabilities; (iv) patients with Axis I disorders and intellectual disabilities. Seventy-one patients (12.9%) had Axis I psychiatric disorders, 245 had only intellectual disability (44.6%) and 33 patients (6%) had an Axis I psychiatric disorder in addition to intellectual disability (Figure 4).

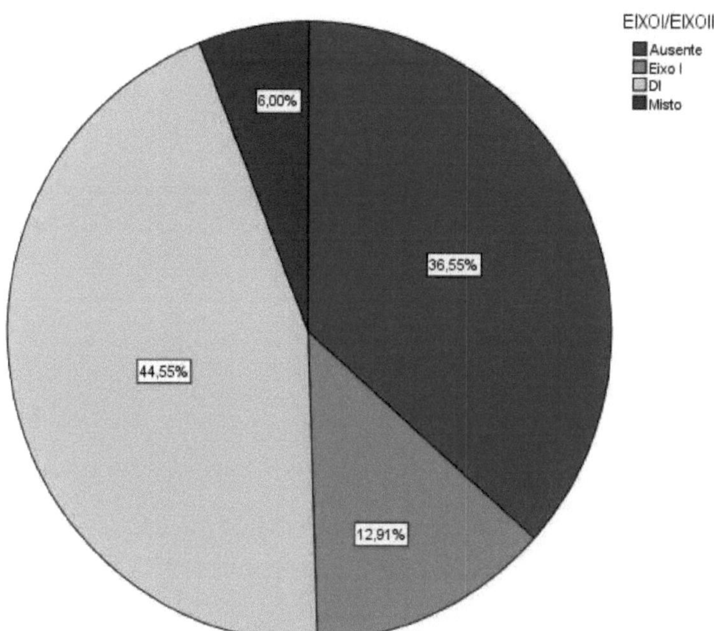

Figure 4 - Frequency of Axis I and II psychiatric comorbidities in patients with cerebral palsy. *Legend: ID*: intellectual disability.

Other frequent psychiatric comorbidities were anxiety disorders (17 patients - 3.1%), behavioural disorders (23 patients - 3.2%), attention deficit hyperactivity disorder (17 patients - 3%), autistic spectrum disorder (33 patients - 6%) and depression (seven patients - 1.3%). Four patients (0.7%) had some other psychiatric disorder (two patients with oppositional defiant disorder, one with psychosis and one with dissociative disorder). Four patients (0.7%) fulfilled diagnostic criteria for more than one Axis I psychiatric disorder (i.e. Mixed) (Figure 5).

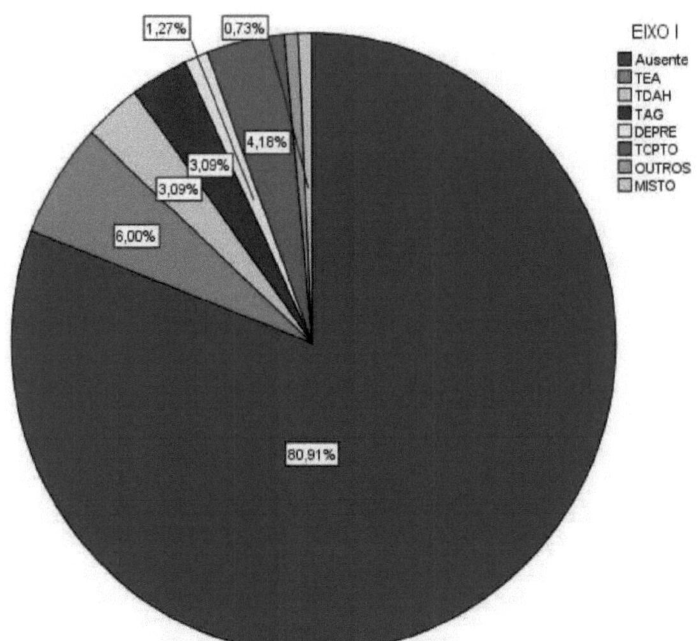

Figure 5 - Frequency of Axis I psychiatric comorbidities in patients with cerebral palsy. *Legend:* ASD: autistic spectrum disorder; ADHD: attention deficit hyperactivity disorder; GAD: generalised anxiety disorder; DEPRE: depression; TCPTO: behavioural disorder.

There was no statistically significant difference between the groups of patients with psychiatric comorbidities (i.e. ASD and ADHD) and control patients when considering the type of CP (ASD vs CONT x^2 =0.00, p=1.000; ADHD vs CONT x^2 =6.26, p=0.180). Table 12 shows the distribution of patients with CP according to the presence of a psychiatric comorbidity and the type of CP.

Table 12 - Distribution of patients with CP according to the presence of a psychiatric comorbidity and the type of CP.

Type of PC	Group		
	TEA	ADHD	Controls
HEMI	8	6	8
Diparetic	18	8	18
Ataxic	1	0	0
COREO	0	1	1
TETRA	6	0	6

Caption: Diparetic: spastic diparetic; HEMI: spastic hemiparetic; COREO: choreoathetoid; ASD: autistic spectrum disorder; ADHD: attention deficit hyperactivity disorder.

5. *Exploring ASD and epilepsy*

We explored the presence of epilepsy in the group of subjects with Autism Spectrum Disorder. The frequency of cases of patients with ASD and epilepsy is higher than the frequency observed in patients who do not have any Axis I psychiatric comorbidity (x2=4.75, p=0.029). The relative risk of having epilepsy in the ASD group was 2.23. On the other hand, the frequency of patients with ASD is similar to the frequency of patients without an Axis I psychiatric disorder and intellectual disability (x2=0.99, p=0.320).

Table 13 - Frequency of epilepsy in patients with and without ASD.

	TEA		
	Absent	TEA	Total
Missing PPE	237	24	261
PPE	209	9	218
Total	446	33	479

Caption-, ASD: autistic spectrum disorder; EPI: epilepsy.

Table 14 - Frequency of intellectual disability in patients with and without ASD.

		TEA		
		Absent	TEA	Total
DI	Absent	202	12	214
	DI	244	21	265
Total		446	33	479

Caption: ASD: autistic spectrum disorder; ID: intellectual disability.

5. *Exploring PPE and PC/level*

As for the classification of cerebral palsy in patients with epilepsy, 218 patients (92.4%) had the spastic form, 40 (16.8%) spastic diparetic, 137 (57.5%) spastic tetraparetic and 41 (18.1%) spastic hemiparetic (23 on the right and 18 on the left). The choreoathetoid form was observed in 13 (5.5%) patients, in one (0.4%) the form was ataxic and six (2.5%) patients had a mixed form (spastic associated with choreoathetoid) (Figure 6).

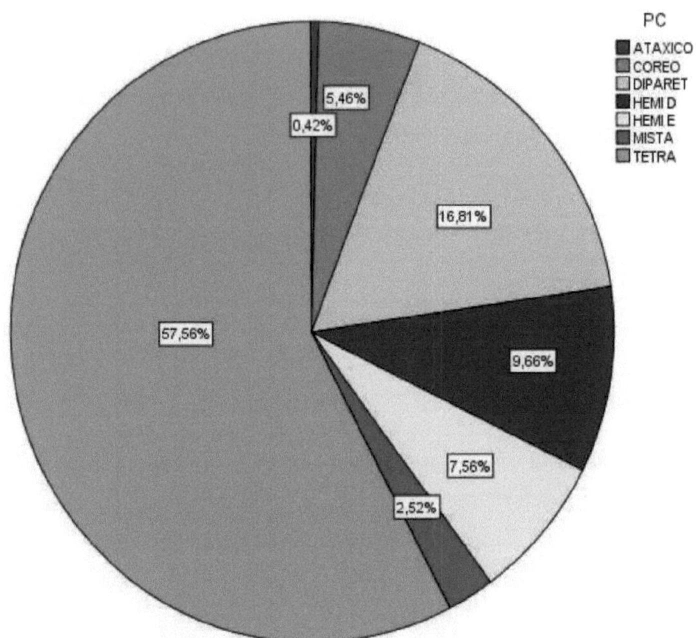

Figure 6 - Frequency of clinical forms in patients with epilepsy.
Key-, Diparetic: spastic diparetic; TETRA: spastic tetraparetic; HEMI: spastic hemiparetic; D: right; E: left; COREO: choreoathetoid.

When the association between motor level and cerebral palsy classification in patients with epilepsy was checked, the following distribution was observed, as shown in Table 15.

Table 15 - Distribution of subjects with epilepsy according to the type of cerebral palsy and their motor level.

	LEVEL					Total
	I	II	III	IV	V	
ATXIC PC	1 (100%)	0	0	0	0	1
COREO	1 (7,7%)	1 (7,7%)	2(15,4%)	2(15,4%)	7 (53,8%)	13
Diparetic	7(17,5%)	8 (20%)	11 (27,5%)	11 (27,5%)	3 (7,5%)	40
HEMI D	15 (65,2%)	4(17,4%)	2 (8,7%)	2 (8,7%)	0	23
HEMI E	8 (44,4%)	4 (22,2%)	4 (22,2%)	2(11,1%)	0	18
MIXED	0	0	1 (16,7%)	0	5 (83,3%)	6
TETRA	0	0	10(7,3%)	48 (35%)	79 (57,7%)	137
Total	32	17	30	65	94	238

Key: Diparetic: spastic diparetic; TETRA: spastic tetraparetic; HEMI: spastic hemiparetic; D: right; E: left; COREO: choreoathetoid.

7. Exploring functionality and psychiatric disorder Axis I

An exploratory analysis was carried out to check the impact of the presence of a psychiatric comorbidity on the functionality of patients with CP. To this end, the CGAS scale was applied to patients diagnosed with ASD and ADHD and their scores were compared with those of control subjects with CP but no psychiatric diagnosis. Patients with moderate/severe intellectual disability were excluded from this sub-analysis.

The ASD group consisted of 12 patients (eight men [66.7%] and four women [33.3%]) with a mean age of 7.75 years (±4.09). In this group, three (25%) patients had spastic hemiparetic CP and nine (75%) had spastic diparetic CP. As for motor level, eight (66.7%) patients could be classified as level I, three (25%) patients were level II and one (8.3%) was level III.

The ADHD group consisted of 15 patients (13 males [86.7%] and two females [13.3%]) with a mean age of 8.93 years (±2.22). In this group, six (40%) patients had spastic hemiparetic CP, eight (53.3%) were spastic diparetic and one (6.7%) was choreoathetoid. As for motor level, 10 (66.7%) patients could be classified as level I, two (13.3%) patients were level II and three (20%) were level III.

Finally, the Control group consisted of 19 patients (13 men [68.4%] and six women [31.6%]) with a mean age of 5.95 years (±4.05). Five (26.3%) patients had spastic hemiparetic CP, 13 (68.4%) had spastic diparetic CP and one (5.3%) had ataxic CP. Eleven (57.9%) patients could be classified as level I, seven (36.8%) as level II and one (5.3%) as level III.

Considering the demographic factors, it was observed that the groups had a similar distribution of individuals in relation to the following factors: gender (x^2 =1.8; p=0.389), type of CP (x^2 =4.7; p=0.584) and level of CP (x^2 =3.7; p=0.450). However, a significant difference between the groups was observed in relation to the participants' age (x^2 =7.78; p=0.020). The ADHD patients were older than the ASD participants (Z=-2.48; p=0.013) and than the control subjects (Z=-2.35; p=0.019).

The presence of a psychiatric disorder had a significant impact on the perceived functionality of children with CP (x^2 =27.53; p<0.001). Patients with ASD and ADHD had lower scores on the CGAS than their peers without a psychiatric disorder (Z=-3.9; p<0.001 and Z=-4.8; p<0.001, respectively). ASD/ADHD patients did not differ in their CGAS scores (Z=-0.7; p=0.498) (Table 16 and Figure 7).

Table 16 - Impact of the presence of a psychiatric comorbidity and the participants' quality of life.

	TEA Mean (SD)	ADHD Mean (SD)	Controls Mean (SD)	Kruskall-Wallis Test	P
CGAS	55,83 (11,77)[a]	55,33 (9,90)[b]	88,43 (11,19)	27,53	<0,001

Caption'. CGAS: Children's Global Assessment Scale; ASD: autism spectrum disorder; ADHD: attention deficit hyperactivity disorder;[a] ASD < Controls, Mann-Whitney Test;[b] ADHD < Controls, Mann-Whitney Test.

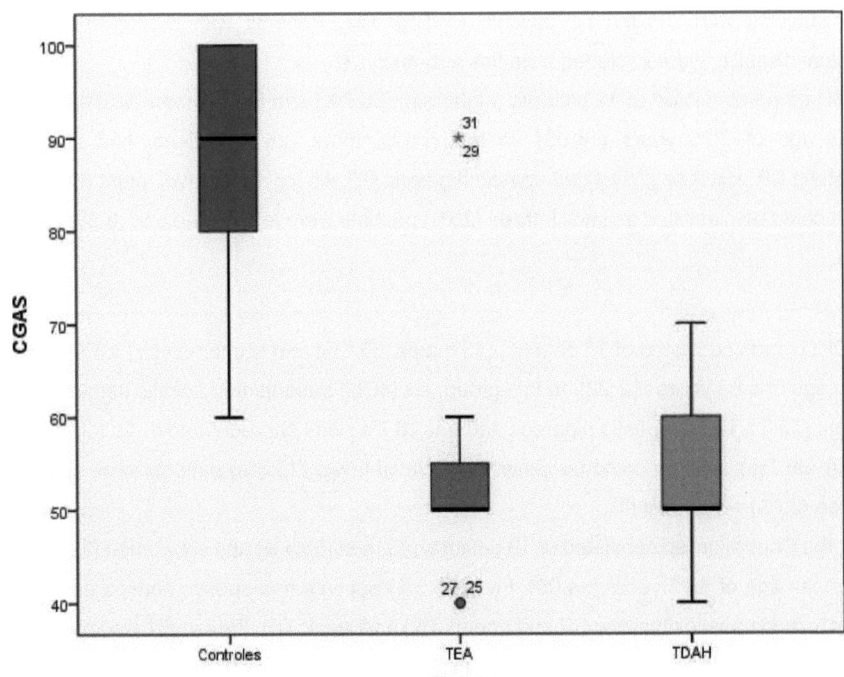

Figure 7 - CGAS scores of patients with CP, divided according to the type of associated psychiatric disorder. There was no statistically significant difference ($x2=4.69$; $p=0.584$) between the groups of patients with psychiatric comorbidities (i.e. ASD and ADHD) and control patients, considering the type of CP. Table 17 shows the distribution of patients with CP according to the presence of a psychiatric comorbidity and the type of CP.

Table 17 - Distribution of patients with CP according to the presence of a psychiatric comorbidity and the type of CP.

	Group		
Type of PC	**TEA**	**ADHD**	**Controls**
HEMI	5	3	6
DIPARET	13	9	8
ATXIC	1	0	0
COREO	0	0	1

Key-, DIPARET: spastic diparetic; HEMI: spastic hemiparetic; COREO: choreoathetoid; ASD: autistic spectrum disorder; ADHD: attention deficit hyperactivity disorder.

CHAPTER 5

DISCUSSION

Nothing belongs to you more than your dreams.

-Friedrich Nietzsche

Although described since the 19th century and relatively well known as a nosological entity, cerebral palsy has been little studied today, especially in relation to the comorbidities that accompany it. CP is not a single entity; it has multiple presentations and multiple variables (Foster, 2010). Previous classifications and definitions have not given due importance to the non-motor impairment of neurological development, performance and behavioural changes that usually accompany CP, nor to the progression of musculoskeletal difficulties that often occurs with advancing age (Rosembaun, 2007).

This work was born out of the author's perception that the diagnosis of psychiatric conditions in children with CP is left in the background, even in tertiary rehabilitation centres, and that complaints relating to these clinical situations are frequent and lead to a significant adaptive impact; and finally, that when the diagnosis is made, there is relief on the part of family members and the child themselves, possibly because there is an explanation for the complaints presented.

Regarding the distribution of the clinical forms of cerebral palsy, our sample is in line with the literature, with the spastic form being the most common, with around 90% of cases, with a higher frequency of the spastic diparetic and tetraparetic forms, followed by the choreoathetoid and mixed forms. There were no cases of the hypotonic form in this sample, which is the least prevalent, also according to the literature (Agarwal & Verma, 2012; Legault *et al,* 2011). There was also no difference in terms of gender.

Although it was not the aim of this study to study the occurrence of epilepsy in this population, given that this is a neurological disease, we found that 43.2 per cent of our patients had this association, and it was more frequent in the spastic tetraparetic form, which is the most clinically severe and where all the studies point to a higher occurrence of other associated clinical situations.

Furthermore, our study was carried out in a tertiary rehabilitation centre and not in an epilepsy centre, so it was not possible to homogenise our sample for the diagnosis of the epileptic syndrome presented, since most of the patients had their electroencephalograms carried out in different locations and with different time specifications and different doctors assessing the tests.

Even so, we can conclude that, in our sample, epilepsy was not a risk factor for psychiatric comorbidities, except for intellectual disability. This finding is explained by the greater severity of the patients with epilepsy in this study.

The presence of an epileptic syndrome was more frequent in patients with spastic forms of CP, however, when we separated our patients according to motor level and clinical form of CP, we obtained few patients in each group, and no statistical difference could be noted between the groups, although we could note a trend towards a greater presence of epilepsy the more severe the motor condition, both in clinical form and motor level. These data are in line with the literature and alert us to the need to actively investigate the presence of epileptic syndromes, especially in the most motorically severe subjects, as the seizure may not be noticed by family members.

CP has traditionally been seen as a motor control disorder, and although this definition is currently being questioned, its therapeutic approach continues to prioritise motor aspects. Treatable psychiatric syndromes in this population have been a neglected area of study (Rosenbaum, 2007; Foster *etal.,* 2010).

A higher prevalence of psychiatric problems is found in patients with CP when compared to control groups, but most studies are carried out using scales applied to parents and carers and with very varied methodology, making it very difficult to homogenise the findings and conclusions. In our study, more than half (61.2%) of our patients presented criteria for the diagnosis of some psychiatric comorbidity in the screening scale applied (PSC) and this figure is in line with the data in the literature (Bjorgaas, Hysing, & Elgen, 2012;

Bjorgaas *et al,* 2013; Brossard-Racine *et aL,* 2012; Foster *et al,* 2010; Goodman & Graham, 1996; Parkes *etal.,* 2008; Tilton & Delgado, 2011).

Although 44.55% of these patients had intellectual disability as a diagnosis, around 13% of the subjects were diagnosed with Axis I psychiatric disorders, without the presence of LD, and 6% had Axis I disorders associated with LD. These figures indicate the need to improve our diagnostic arsenal for children and adolescents with CP that goes beyond ID.

It is important to emphasise that the presence of intellectual disability is a psychiatric risk factor (Streeme & Diseth, 2000). Patients with ID have fewer psychological protection mechanisms and need more family and professional support.

The PSC scale, validated in Brazil by Muzzolon, Cat and Santos (2013), proved to be easy to apply and very sensitive for this population. All the patients who scored as a positive risk had a psychiatric diagnosis confirmed later on clinical examination.

Behavioural disorders were observed in 3.2% of our cases. This figure is lower than that observed in some studies (Brossard-Racine *et al*, 2012; Bjorgaas *et aL,* 2013), probably due to methodological differences. We considered behavioural disorders to be patients whose main complaint was linked to behaviour, without the presence of another psychiatric diagnosis to explain these alterations, such as ASD or ADHD.

Another issue to think about is that almost half of our patients (47.45%) had motor level IV or V, i.e. they are severely affected individuals from a motor point of view, with little functionality, high dependency and, consequently, little cognitive resources, including for behavioural disorders.

In these cases, the family often adapts to the needs of a totally dependent child and begins to meet all the patient's demands without too much opposition, which avoids behavioural or conduct problems, as they are not exposed to frustrations.

Managing children and adolescents with behavioural changes is a stress factor for families and schools (Blacher & Baker, 2007), so making the right diagnosis and intervention in these cases is of fundamental importance for the best adaptation of the patient and their family.

The negative impact of psychiatric disorders can be seen not only in the patient's life but also in that of their family. This family impact already exists because of the physical disability and, when added to the psychiatric issue, it makes family and community life much worse. In this study, the family impact was not actively researched, but subjective reports show its presence in practically all cases, especially in the presence of an associated psychiatric diagnosis. Therefore, mental health services should routinely be part of the follow-up of patients with cerebral palsy, aiming not only to treat the patient, but also to provide support and psychoeducation for family members and the school (Bjorgaas *et al.,* 2012).

The correct identification and management of these comorbidities is necessary to provide these children with more comprehensive care for their condition (Tilton & Delgado, 2011).

To this end, staff at rehabilitation centres caring for patients with CP must be prepared to recognise and manage patients' behavioural and emotional alterations. The presence of screening and psychiatric diagnostic scales, which are objective and easy to use, should be part of the investigative arsenal of every neurological rehabilitation centre. This study demonstrates that the serial application of a screening scale, with subsequent objective examination of positive patients, changes the whole understanding of that patient and the difficulties underlying the physical disability, alerting us to the existence of situations that require a differentiated approach.

Internalising disorders, such as depression and anxiety, are very difficult to diagnose in childhood and even more so in patients with CP (Blackman & Conaway, 2014). In our sample, we observed a relatively low frequency of these disorders when compared to the literature (3.1% for anxiety and 1.3% for depression), possibly due to a sample bias, where in view of the severity of the motor and neurological condition presented, these disorders are often minimised (Levy-Zaks *et al.,* 2014).

Another factor that may explain the low occurrence of these disorders in our population is the fact that the screening scale was carried out with the main caregiver, who, even in normal populations, tends to minimise the signs and symptoms of internalising disorders in the paediatric age group (Blackman & Conaway, 2014).

The presence of pain and/or surgical procedures is also an important factor that increases the frequency of internalising disorders (Yamaguchi *et al.,* 2004). All the patients in this sample were outpatients and were not pre- or post-operative, which may also explain the low frequency of these disorders.

In any case, actively investigating the presence of internalising disorders in children and adolescents with cerebral palsy should be part of the diagnostic and therapeutic arsenal of specialised centres. Although its frequency may be lower than that of the normal population (a fact that still requires further investigation), it is important to keep an eye out for the occurrence of this clinical situation in this population, since the therapeutic approach to this association improves not only the patient's quality of life but also helps with their motor rehabilitation.

Due to the low number of patients diagnosed with Anxiety Disorders / Depression, it was not possible to identify a predominant clinical form of CP. However, we did not observe the presence of internalising disorders in patients with ILD, warning that this diagnosis should be effectively considered in patients with good cognitive performance.

Attention Deficit Hyperactivity Disorder was observed in 3%, a lower rate than that observed in the general population (Faraone *et al.,* 2003) and with a higher occurrence in boys, which is in line with the literature.

This lower figure can be explained by the fact that we didn't consider patients with moderate to severe intellectual disabilities to be diagnosed with ADHD. When patients with LD are excluded, the occurrence of the disorder rises to 6.3 per cent, which is in line with the general literature, but still below the casuistry in patients with CP, which speaks of a 10 to 50 per cent frequency of ADHD in this group (Goodman & Graham, 1996; Parkes *etal.,* 2008; Bjorgaas, Hysing, *et al.* 2012; Bjorgaas *et al.,* 2014).

However, these studies were carried out using screening scales with family members, which may increase the rate of diagnosis, as well as not excluding patients with ID who present symptoms compatible with ADHD secondary to cognitive deficits. Psychomotor agitation and short attention spans in patients with intellectual disabilities were considered secondary to cognitive impairment and not ADHD in this study.

In addition, the signs and symptoms scale for ADHD (SNAP IV) was applied in at least two environments (family and school or therapy) and the diagnosis was only considered when there was agreement between the two applications, confirmed by clinical assessment based on the DSM-5.

In a Brazilian study, Coutinho, Mattos, Schmitz, Fortes, & Borges (2009) showed that agreement on the diagnosis between parents and teachers is moderate and occurs in just over half of the cases (59.09 per cent), so applying scales only to family members may reveal a higher prevalence, as observed in these studies.

ADHD in itself is a disorder with a high level of family and academic impact. Thinking about this association in patients with CP is fundamental for better social and, especially, academic inclusion.

Because of the peculiarities observed in this group of patients, actively investigating the occurrence of this disorder should be carried out carefully and preferably by a multidisciplinary team.

Autism spectrum disorders can currently be understood as the expression of atypical brain development, resulting in more or less widespread dysfunctions, widely distributed in the neural network. In this context, it is to be expected that children with cerebral palsy whose development is based on a damaged nervous system will have a higher frequency of ASD.

Due to their motor alterations, children with CP often have less spontaneous contact with the environment and their potential for social interaction is lower when compared to other children. Cailies, Hody and Calmus (2012), studying 20 subjects with CP and 20 controls, observed that individuals with CP have greater difficulties with theory of mind and understanding irony. We did not investigate separate aspects within the autism spectrum, however part of the findings of adaptive difficulties, such as difficulty understanding irony and putting oneself in another person's shoes, in children with ASD and CP, are due to these alterations in theory of mind and were not observed in children with CP alone.

Kilincast and Mukaddes (2008), in a review of this association, observed three groups of studies: 1) studies focused on the occurrence of medical disorders in children with ASD; 2) a group where the occurrence of ASD and CP is related to other situations, such as visual impairment and hydrocephalus; and 3) a group that evaluates the presence of ASD in children with CP. The smallest number of studies was found in this group, showing that the population of children with CP is very little studied in relation to this comorbidity.

Our study assessed individuals with cerebral palsy, actively investigating the presence of psychiatric comorbidities, and found a 6% frequency of ASD, which is around six times higher than the frequency of ASD in the general population. Kilincaslan and Mukaddes (2008) found a 15% prevalence of ASD in their sample and the type of CP (tetra- and hemiplegic), the presence of epilepsy and the intellectual level were the relevant differences between the groups. We did not observe any significant differences between the clinical forms of CP, as did Kirby *et al.* (2011). On the other hand, in our sample the presence of ASD was significantly higher in patients with epilepsy.

Also according to the literature, in our group there was a greater occurrence of ASD in subjects with LD, but this difference was not statistically significant.

When we compared subjects with an association of ASD or ADHD, without moderate to severe intellectual disability, with subjects with CP without comorbidities, we observed a predominance in levels I, II and III, corroborating the idea that subjects with less motor impairment have better intellectual function, but have other psychiatric disorders.

We also found a statistically significant difference in the overall functioning of these individuals, i.e. the presence of a psychiatric disorder impaired their overall functioning more than the presence of a physical disability. This data alerts us to the urgent need to implement systematised protocols for psychiatric diagnosis in people with cerebral palsy. In this group, there was also no predominance of the clinical form of CP.

The most frequent comorbidity found was intellectual disability, observed in 44.5% of patients, with no difference in relation to gender, which differs from studies on ID without CP, where the prevalence is higher in boys (Lai *et al.*, 2012; Patterson & Zoghbi, 2003). This occurrence is also in line with that found in the literature (Andersen *et al.*, 2008; Himmelmann *et al.*, 2006; Huang, Tseng, Chen, Shieh, & Lu, 2013; Koman *et al.*, 2004; Singhi & Saini, 2013; Tan *et al.*, 2014). This association causes major limitations in the lives of children with CP and their carers, and their diagnosis is not actively carried out (Raina *et al.*, 2005). This situation implies both not diagnosing children with SLD and subjectively inferring this diagnosis in patients with preserved cognition but with other conditions, such as dysarthria and dyspraxia. Few services routinely screen and research cognitive aspects in children with cerebral palsy using objective tests.

Delacy and Reid (2016) also point out an important issue in the cognitive assessment of these individuals. Many of them have difficulty answering standardised tests, as most require verbal responses, motor coordination or written responses, which leads to many diagnoses of "probably deficient". We also observed these difficulties and, because of this, all the children were also assessed using an adaptive behaviour scale and taking motor difficulties into account

DL has a higher occurrence in tetra spastic forms of CP (Andersen *et al.*, 2008; Himmelmann *et al.*, 2006). This frequency increases progressively according to motor level, regardless of clinical form (Delacy & Reid, 2016). Our study also found a higher frequency in children with a motor level above III, suggesting that routine assessments of the intellectual aspect should be carried out especially in children with a motor level above III, regardless of the clinical type. The tetra-spastic form, being the most frequent at levels IV and V, was the one with the highest number of LD diagnoses.

Most of these subjects had moderate or severe LD (42.75 per cent and 40.63 per cent, respectively). In this group, the diagnosis is easier to make, but 16.6% had mild LD, where the diagnosis can be confused with other disorders, especially ADHD. In these children, school and behavioural complaints predominated.

Diagnosing intellectual disability in patients with CP is important not only from an academic and rehabilitation point of view, but also in relation to the quality of life of these families, since ASD, sensory impairments and LD are identified as having the greatest negative impact on family members (Boulet *etal.,* 2009; Bostrõm *etal.,* 2010).

Although LD is one of the most frequent comorbidities in CP and plays a significant role in the overall functional impact of these patients, its diagnosis has been underappreciated and little taken into account in the rehabilitation of these patients, as well as in their school, social and professional inclusion. If we consider that almost half of our patients have LD associated with CP, rehabilitation services for people with cerebral palsy must include cognitive rehabilitation.

Intellectual disability is more important for social participation than the GMFCS level and one of the main factors for a good evolution of patients with CP (Liptak & Accardo, 2004; Tan *et aL,* 2014). This data, coupled with the high frequency of this diagnosis in the group in question, again leads us to question the rehabilitation models currently used, where the cognitive issue, which has the greatest functional impact, is left in the background.

Active research into comorbidities should be routine practice within tertiary rehabilitation centres.

The presence of mental health professionals in physical rehabilitation centres is not routine in our country, but our results point to the urgent need for this technical apparatus for a better therapeutic outcome.

Knowing the impact of the association of motor and cognitive conditions on the lives of the family and the child is of fundamental importance if we are to think of CP not as an entity, but as a heterogeneous set of clinical situations that impact on the life of the patient and their environment, and the inclusion of mental health in rehabilitation protocols is an important step towards a better prognosis and improved functionality and adaptation of these patients.

Finally, it is worth emphasising that intellectual disability must also be carefully observed and studied in the treatment of these children, and its accurate and correct diagnosis must be actively sought.

Thinking about the rehabilitation of patients with CP must go beyond the physical objectives and look with the same attention at the emotional, behavioural, academic and social aspects.

CHAPTER 6

CONCLUSIONS

A mind that is open to a new idea will never return to its original size.
-Albert Einstein

The occurrence of psychiatric disorders in patients with CP is higher than in the general population. Regardless of the clinical form and motor level, the investigation of psychiatric conditions should be actively carried out in this population. The more severe the patient, the greater the occurrence of comorbidities, including epilepsy, which was more frequent in patients with ASD.

The presence of psychiatric disorders worsens the functionality and, consequently, the quality of life of these children and their families.

Future studies are needed, especially to elucidate more clearly the relationship between clinical forms and the occurrence of mental disorders.

CHAPTER 7

REFERENCES

Every force is weak if it is not united.

-Jean de La Fontaine

Agarwal, A., & Verma, I. (2012). Cerebral palsy in children: an overview. *J Clin Orthop Trauma, 3*, 77-81. doi: 10.1016/j.jcot.2012.09.001

Andersen, G. L., Irgens, L. M., Haagaas, I., Skranes, J. S., Meberg, A. E., & Vik, T. (2008). Cerebral palsy in Norway: prevalence, subtypes and severity. *Eur J Paediatr Neurol, 12(1)*, 4-13. doi: 10.1016/j.ejpn.2007.05.001

(2013) DSM - 5 - *Diagnostic and Statistical Manual of Mental Disorders* (5ª ed.). Arlington, VA: American Psychiatric Publishing

Assumpção Jr, F. B. (2000). Childhood Autism. In A. C. M. Pimentel (Ed.), (Vol. 22, pp. 37-39).

Assumpção Júnior, F. B., Gonçalves, J. D. M., Cuccolichio, S., Amorim, L. C. D., Rego, F., Gomes, C., & Falcão, M. S. (2008). Autistic Traits Assessment Scale (ATA): second validity study / Scale for the assessment of Autistic Behaviour (ATA). *Med e Reab, 27(2)*, 41-44.

Bass, N. (1999). Cerebral palsy and neurodegenerative disease. *Curr Opin Pediatr, 11(6)*, 504- 507.

Bax, M., Goldstein, M., Rosenbaum, P., Leviton, A., Paneth, N., Dan, B., Jacobsson, B. & Damiano, D. (2005). Proposed definition and classification of cerebral palsy, April 2005. *Dev Med Child Neurol, 47(8)*, 571-576.

Biederman, J. (2005). Attention-deficit/hyperactivity disorder: a selective overview. *Biol Psychiatry, 57(11)*, 1215-1220. doi: 10.1016/j.biopsych.2004.10.020

Binnie, C. D., & Marston, D. (1992). Cognitive correlates of interictal discharges. *Epilepsia, 33 Suppl 6*, S11-17.

Birmaher, B., Brent, D., Bernet, W., Bukstein, O., Walter, H., Benson, R. S., Chrisman, A., Farchione, T., Greenhill, L., Hamilton, J., Keable, H., Kinlan, J., Schoettle, U., Stock, S., Ptakowski, K. K. & Medicus, J. (2007). Practice parameter for the assessment and treatment of children and adolescents with depressive disorders. *J Am Acad Child Adolesc Psychiatry, 46(11)*, 1503-1526. doi: 10.1097/chi.0b013e318145ae1c

Bjorgaas, H. M., Elgen, I., Boe, T., & Hysing, M. (2013). Mental health in children with cerebral palsy: does screening capture the complexity? *ScientificWorldJournal, 3*. doi: 10.1155/2013/468402

Bjorgaas, H. M., Hysing, M., & Elgen, I. (2012). Psychiatric disorders among children with cerebral palsy at school starting age. *Res Dev Disabil, 33(4)*, 1287-1293. doi: 10.1016/j.ridd.2012.02.024

Blacher, J., & Baker, B. L. (2007). Positive impact of intellectual disability on families. *Am J Ment Retard, 112(5)*, 330-348. doi: 10.1352/0895-8017(2007)112[0330:PIOIDO]2.0.CG;2

Blackman, J. A., & Conaway, M. R. (2014). Adolescents with cerebral palsy: transitioning to adult health care services. *Clin Pediatr (Phila), 53(4)*, 356-363. doi: 10.1177/0009922813510203

Bostrõm, P., Broberg, M., & Hwang, C. P. (2010). Different, difficult or distinct? Mothers' and fathers' perceptions of temperament in children with and without intellectual disabilities. *J Intellect Disabil Res, 54(9)*, 806-819. doi: 10.1111/j.1365-2788.2010.01309.x

Boulet, S. L., Boyle, C. A., & Schieve, L. A. (2009). Health care use and health and functional impact of developmental disabilities among US children, 1997-2005. *Arch Pediatr Adolesc Med, 163(1)*, 19-26. doi: 10.1001/archpediatrics.2008.506

Brand-Gothelf, A., Yoeli-Bligh, N., Gilboa-Schechtman, E., Benaroya-Milshtein, N., & Apter, A. (2014). Perceptions of self, mother and family and behaviour of prepubertal depressed children. *Eur Psychiatry.* doi: 10.1016/j.eurpsy.2014.05.005

Brossard-Racine, M., Hall, N., Majnemer, A., Shevell, M. I., Law, M., Poulin, C., & Rosenbaum, P. (2012). Behavioural problems in school age children with cerebral palsy. *Eur J Paediatr Neurol, 16(1)*, 35-41. doi: http://dx.doi.Org/10.1016/j.ejpn.2011.10.001

Caillies, S., Hody, A. & Calmus, A. (2012) Theory of mind and irony comprehension in children with cerebral palsy. *Res Dev Disabil, 33(5)*, 1380-1388.

Cartwright-Hatton, S., McNicol, K., & Doubleday, E. (2006). Anxiety in a neglected population: prevalence of anxiety disorders in pre-adolescent children. *Clin Psychol Rev, 26(7)*, 817- 833. doi: 10.1016/j.cpr.2005.12.002

Costa, M. I., & Nunesmaia, H. G. (1998). [Genetic and clinicai diagnosis of infantile autism], *Arq Neuropsiquiatr, 56(1)*, 24-31.

Costello, E. J., Costello, A. J., Edelbrock, C., Bums, B. J., Dulcan, M. K., Brent, D. & Janiszewski, S. (1988) Psychiatric Disorders in Paediatric Primary Care: Prevalence and Risk Factors. *Arch Gen Psychiatry, 45(12)*:1107-1116.

Coutinho, G., Mattos, P., Schmitz, M., Fortes, D. & Borges, M. (2009). Agreement rates between parents' and teachers' reports on ADHD symptomatology: findings from a Brazilian clinicai sample. *Archives of Clinicai Psychiatry, 36(3)*, 97-100.

Delacy, M. J. & Reid, S. M. (2016). Profile of associated impairments at age 5 years in Australia by cerebral palsy subtype and Gross Motor Function Classification System levei for birth years 1996 to 2005. *Dev Med Child Neurol, 58 (2)*, 50-56.

Desai, M. II., Divan, G., Wertz, F. J., & Patel, V. (2012). The discovery of autism: Indian parents' experiences of caring for their child with an autism spectrum disorder. *Transcult Psychiatry, 49(3-4)*, 613-637. doi: 10.1177/1363461512447139

Diament, A. (1996). Chronic encephalopathy in childhood (cerebral palsy). In A. Diament & S. Cypel (Eds.), *Neurologia Infantil* (3ª ed., pp. 781-798). São Paulo: Ed. Atheneu.

Faraone, S. V., Sergeant, J., Gillberg, C., & Biederman, J. (2003). The worldwide prevalence of ADHD: is it an American condition? *World Psychiatry, 2(2)*, 104-113.

Fleitlich-Bilyk, B. & Goodman, R. (2004). Prevalence of Child and Adolescent Psychiatric Disorders in Southeast Brazil. *J Am Acad Child Adolesc Psychiatry, 43(6)*, 727-734.

Fombonne, E. (2009). Epidemiology of pervasive developmental disorders. *Paediatr Res, 65(6)*, 591-598.

Foster, T., Rai, A. I. K., Weller, R. A., Dixon, T. A., & Weller, E. B. (2010). Psychiatric Complications in Cerebral Palsy. *Curr Psychiatry Rep, 12(2)*, 116-121. doi: 10.1007/sl 1920-010-0096-8

Gabis, L., Pomeroy, J., & Andriola, M. R. (2005). Autism and epilepsy: cause, consequence, comorbidity, or coincidence? *Epilepsy Behav, 7(4)*, 652-656. doi: 10.1016/j.yebeh.2005.08.008

Gadia, C. A., Tuchman, R., & Rotta, N. T. (2004). [Autism and pervasive developmental disorders]. *J Pediatr (Rio J.), 80(2 Suppl)*, S83-94.

Gillberg, C. (1990). Autism and Pervasive Developmental Disorders. *J Child Psychol Psychiatry, 37*,99-119.

Goodman, R. (1998). The longitudinal stability of psychiatric problems in children with hemiplegia. *J Child Psychol Psychiatry, 39(3)*, 347-354.

Goodman, R., & Graham, P. (1996). Psychiatric problems in children with hemiplegia: cross sectional epidemiological survey. *BMJ, 372(7038)*, 1065-1069.

Graham, P. & Rutter, M. (1968). Organic Brain Dysfunction and Child Psychiatric Disorder. *Br Med J,3*, 695-700.

Himmelmann, K., Beckung, E., Hagberg, G., & Uvebrant, P. (2006). Gross and fine motor function and accompanying impairments in cerebral palsy. *Dev Med Child Neurol, 48(6)*, 417-423. doi: 10.1017/S0012162206000922

Huang, C. Y., Tseng, M. H., Chen, K. L., Shieh, J. Y., & Lu, L. (2013). Detemninants of school activity performance in children with cerebral palsy: a multidimensional approach using the ICF-CY as a framework. *Res Dev Disabil,* 34(11), 4025-4033. doi: 10.1016/j.ridd.2013.08.022

Katz, G., & Lazcano-Ponce, E. (2008). Intellectual disability: definition, etiological factors, classification, diagnosis, treatment and prognosis. *Salud Publica Mex, 50 Suppl 2,* s132- 141.

Kilincaslan, A., & Mukaddes, N. M. (2009). Pervasive developmental disorders in individuals with cerebral palsy. *Dev Med Child Neurol, 51(4),* 289-294. doi: 10.1111/j.1469-8749.2008.03171.x

Kirby, S. R., Wingate, M. S., Braun, K. N., Doemberg, N. S., Ameson, C. L., Benedict, R. E., Mulvihill, B., Durkin, M. S., Fitzgerald, R. T., Maenner, M. J., Patz, J. A. & Yeargin-Allsopp, M. (2011). Prevalence and functioning of children with cerebral palsy in four areas of the United States in 2006: a report from the Autism and Developmental Disabilities Monitoring Network. *Res Dev Disabil,* 32(2):462-469.

Koman, L. A., Smith, B. P., & Shilt, J. S. (2004). Cerebral palsy. *Lancet,* 363(9421), 1619-1631. doi: 10.1016/S0140-6736(04)16207-7

Lagault, G., Shevell, M. I. & Dagenais, L. (2011). Predicting Comorbidities With Neuroimaging in Children With Cerebral Palsy. *Paediatr Neurol, 45,* 229-232.

Lai, D. C., Tseng, Y.C., Hou Y.M. & Guo, H.R. (2012). Genderand geographic differences in the prevalence of intellectual disability in children: analysis of data from the national disability registry of Taiwan. *Res Dev Disabil,* 33(6),2301-2017.

Lenoir, P., Bodier, C., Desombre, H., Malvy, J., Abert, B., Ould Taleb, M., & Sauvage, D. (2009). [Prevalence of pervasive developmental disorders. A review], *Encephale,* 35(1), 36-42. doi: 10.1016/j.encep.2007.12.011

Levy-Zaks, A., Pollak, Y., & Ben-Pazi, H. (2014). Cerebral palsy risk factors and their impact on psychopathology. *Neurol Res,* 36(1), 92-94. doi: 10.1179/1743132813Y.0000000290

Liptak, G. S. & Accardo, P.J. (2004) Health and Social Outcomes of Children with Cerebral Palsy. *J Paediatr, 145(2),* S36-41.

Mancini, M. C., Fiúza, P. M., Rebelo, J. M., Magalhães, L. C., Coelho, Z. A., Paixao, M. L., Gontijo, A. P. B. & Fonseca, S. T. (2002). Comparison of functional activity performance in normally developing children and children with cerebral palsy. *Arq Neuropsiquiatr,* 60(2-B), 446-452.

Martini, D. R. (1995). Common anxiety disorders in children and adolescents. *Curr Probl Pediatr,* 25(9), 271-280.

Matthews, M., Nigg, J. T. & Fair, D. A. (2014). Attention deficit hyperactivity disorder. *Curr Top Behav Neurosci, 16,* 235 66.

Mattos, P., Serra-Pinhoiro, M. A., Rohde, L. A., & Pinto, D. (2006). Presentation of a Portuguese version for use in Brazil of the MTA-SNAP-IV instrument for assessing symptoms of attention-deficit/hyperactivity disorder and symptoms of oppositional defiant disorder. *Rev Psiquiatr Rio Gd Sul,* 28(3), 290-297.

Michelsen, S. I., Flachs, E. M., Damsgaard, M. T., Parkes, J., Parkinson, K., Rapp, M., Arnaud, C., Nystrand, M., Colver, A., Fauconnier, J., Dickinson, H.O., Marcelli, M. & Uldall, P. (2014). European study of frequency of participation of adolescents with and without cerebral palsy. *Eur J Paediatr Neurol, 18(3),* 282-294.

Muzzolon, S. R., Cat, M. N., & dos Santos, L. H. (2013). Evaluation of the Pediatric Symptom Checklist as a screening tool for the Identification of emotional and psychosocial problems. *Rev Paul Pediatr, 31(3),* 359-365. doi: 10.1590/S0103-05822013000300013

Newman, C. J., 0'Regan, M., & Hensey, O. (2006). Sleep disorders in children with cerebral palsy. *Dev Med Child Neurol, 48(7),* 564-568. doi: 10.1017/S0012162206001198

Palisano, R., Rosenbaum, P., Walter, S., Russell, D., Wood, E., & Galuppi, B. (1997). Development and reliability of a system to classify gross motor function in children with cerebral palsy. *Dev Med Child Neurol,* 39(4), 214-223.

Parkes, J., & McCusker, C. (2008). Common psychological problems in cerebral palsy. *Paediatr Child Health, 18(9),* 427-431. doi: http://dx.doi.Org/10.1016/j.paed.2008.05.012

Parkes, J., White-Koning, M., Dickinson, H. O., Thyen, U., Arnaud, C., Beckung, E., Fauconnier, J., Marcelli, M., McManus, V., Michelsen, S. I., Parkinson, K. & Colver,

A. (2008). Psychological problems in children with cerebral palsy: a cross-sectional European study. *J Child Psychol Psychiatry, 49(4)*, 405-413.

Patterson, M. C. & Zoghbi, H.Y. (2003). Mental retardation: X marks the spot. *Neurology, 6,* 156- 157.

Raina, P., 0'Donnell, M., Rosenbaum, P., Brehaut, J., Walter, S. D., Russell, D., Swinton, M., Zhu, B. & Wood, E. (2005). The health and well-being of caregivers of children with cerebral palsy. *Paediatrics, 115(6)*, e626-636.

Rapin, I. (2002). The autistic-spectrum disorders. *N Engl J Med, 347(5)*, 302-303. doi: 10.1056/NEJMp020062

Rosenbaum, P., Paneth, N., Leviton, A., Goldstein, M., Bax, M., Damiano, D., Dan, B. & Jacobsson, B. (2007). A report: the definition and classification of cerebral palsy (2006). *Dev Med Child Neurol Suppl, 109*, 8-14.

Shaffer, D., Gould, M., Brasic, J., Ambrosini, P., Fisher, P., Bird, H., & Aluwahlia, S. (1983). A children's global assessment scale (CGAS). *Arch Gen Psychiatry, 40,*1228-1231.

Silva, D. B., Pfeifer, L. I., & Funayama, C. A. (2013). Gross Motor Function Classification System Expanded & Revised (GMFCS E & R): reliability between therapists and parents in Brazil. *BrazJPhys Ther, 17(5)*, 458-463. doi: 10.1590/S1413-35552012005000113

Singhi, P., & Saini, A. G. (2013). Changes in the clinical spectrum of cerebral palsy over two decades in North India--an analysis of 1212 cases. *J Trop Pediatr, 59(6)*, 434-440. doi: 10.1093/tropej/fmt035

Sparrow, S. S., Cicchetti, V. D, & Baila D. A. (1984). Vineland adaptive behaviour scales. American Guidance Service: Circle Pines.

Spence, S.H. (1998). A measure of anxiety symptoms among children. *Behav Res Ther, 36(5)*, 545-566.

Spence, S. J., & Schneider, M. T. (2009). The role of epilepsy and epileptiform EEGs in autism spectrum disorders. *Pediatr Res, 65(6)*, 599-606. doi: 10.1203/PDR.0b013e31819e7168

Streeme, P. & Diseth, T. H. (2000). Prevalence of psychiatric diagnoses in children with mental retardation: data from a population-based study. *Dev Med Child Neurol, 42,* 266-270.

Tan, S. S., Wiegerink, D. J., Vos, R. C., Smits, D. W., Voorman, J. M., Twisk, J. W., Ketelaar, M., Roebroek, M. E. & PERRIN study group (2014). Developmental trajectories of social participation in individuals with cerebral palsy: a multicentre longitudinal study. *Dev Med Child Neurol, 56(4)*, 370-377.

Taylor, E. Antecedents of ADHD: a historical account of diagnostic concepts (2011). *Atten Defic Hyperact Disord*, 3(2):69-75.

Tilton, A. & Delgado, M. R. (2011). Paediatric patients with cerebral palsy or other developmental disabilities. *Semin Pediatr Neurol, 18(2)*72-73.

Tuchman, R. F., Rapin, I., & Shinnar, S. (1991). Autistic and dysphasic children. II: Epilepsy. *Pediatrics, 88(6)*, 1219-1225.

Vargus-Adams, J. (2005). Health-related quality of life in childhood cerebral palsy. *Arch Phys Med Rehabil, 86(5)*, 940-945. doi: 10.1016/j.apmr.2004.10.036

Vianna, R. R. A. B., Campos, A. A. & Landeira-Fernandez, J. (2009). Anxiety Disorders in Childhood and Adolescence: A review. *RevBras TerCogn*, 5(1), 46-61

Yamaguchi, R., Nicholson Perry, K., & Hines, M. (2014). Pain, pain anxiety and emotional and behavioural problems in children with cerebral palsy. *Disabil Rehabil, 36(2)*, 125-130. doi: 10.3109/09638288.2013.782356

Zablotsky, B., Black, L. I., Maenner, M. J., Schieve, L. A. & Blumberg, S. J. (2015). Estimated Prevalence of Autism and Other Developmental Disabilities Following Questionnaire Changes in the 2014 National Health Interview Survey. *Natl Health Stat Report,13(Q7)*A- 20.

CHAPTER 8

ANNEXES

ANNEX A - PSC SCALE - *Paediatric Symptom Checklist* **(Muzzolon et al., 2013).**

Symptom checklist		No	Sometimes	Often
01	Complains of pain without a physical cause			
02	Spends most of his time alone			
03	Gets tired easily			
04	He's restless, he won't sit still			
05	Has relationship problems with teachers			
06	Little interest in learning			
07	It acts as if it were driven by a "little motor"			
08	"Dreams a lot during the day			
09	Easily distracted			
10	Afraid to face new situations			
11	Feeling sad or unhappy			
12	He's angry, irritated			
13	You feel abandoned, hopeless			
14	Problems concentrating			
15	Has little interest in having friends			
16	Fighting with other children			
17	Missing school for no reason			
18	Your school grades are falling			
19	Feeling inferior			
20	He consults several doctors, who find nothing			
21	Difficulty sleeping			
22	Is a very worried or tense child			
23	He wants to stay with his parents more than before			
24	Feels like "a bad child"			
25	Taking unnecessary risks			
26	Hurt frequently			
27	He's been less cheerful			
28	Act as if you were younger			
29	Disobeys rules			
30	Has difficulty showing their feelings			
31	Doesn't care about other people's feelings			
32	Teasing, mocking or picking on others			
33	Blaming others for your difficulties			
34	Take objects that don't belong to you			
35	Refuses to share objects			

ANNEX B - ATA - AUTISTIC TRAITS SCALE (Assumpção Júnior et al., 2008).

I. DIFFICULTY IN SOCIAL INTERACTION

The deviation from sociability can range from mild forms, such as a certain negativism and not accepting eye contact, to more serious forms, such as intense isolation.

1 Doesn't smile; 2. Absence of spontaneous approaches; 3. Doesn't seek company;

4 . Constantly seeks his or her own corner (hiding place); 5. Avoids people; 6. Is unable to maintain a social exchange; 7. Intense isolation

II. MANIPULATING THE ENVIRONMENT

The problem of manipulating the environment can be more or less serious, such as not responding to requests and remaining indifferent to the environment. The most common occurrence is the sudden outbursts of temper tantrums, uncontrollable laughter for no reason, all with the aim of being the centre of attention

1. No response to requests; 2. Sudden change of mood; 3. Remains indifferent, expressionless; 4. Compulsive laughter; 5. Tantrums and temporary anger; 6. Motor or verbal excitement (going from one place to another, talking non-stop)

III. USING THE PEOPLE AROUND YOU

His relationship with the adult is almost never interactive, as he usually uses the adult as a means to get what he wants.

1. He uses the adult as an object, leading him to what he wants; 2.The adult serves as a support to achieve what he wants (e.g. he uses the

adult as a support to pick up a biscuit); 3. the adult is the means to fulfil a need that they are unable to fulfil on their own (e.g. tying shoes); 4. if the adult does not respond to their demands, they act by interfering in the adult's behaviour.

IV. RESISTANCE TO CHANGE

Resistance to change can range from irritability to outright refusal.

1. Insistent on keeping to a routine; 2. Great difficulty in accepting facts that alter their routine, such as changes of place, clothing and diet; 3. Resistant to change, persisting in the same response or activity

V. SEARCH FOR A RIGID ORDER

They show a tendency to order everything, and can reach obsessive behaviour, without which they are unable to carry out any activity.

1. Sorting objects according to their own pre-established criteria;
2. it is linked to a spatial order (each thing always in its place); 3. it is linked to a temporal sequence (each thing in its time);
4. it is linked to a person-place correspondence (each person is always in a specific

place)

VI. LACK OF EYE CONTACT. BLANK STARE

Lack of contact can range from a strange look to constant avoidance of visual stimuli

1. Averting direct gazes, not looking you in the eye; 2. Turning your head or gaze when called (looking away); 3. Expressing an empty, lifeless gaze; 4. When you follow stimuli with your eyes, you only do so in a way that's not very good for you.

5. fixates on objects with a peripheral gaze, not a central one; 6. gives the impression of not looking

VII. INEXPRESSIVE MIMICRY

Inexpressive mimicry reveals a lack of non-verbal communication. It can range from a certain expressiveness to a total lack of response.

1. If they speak, they don't use facial, gestural or vocal expressions as often as expected; 2.They don't show an anticipatory reaction; 3.They don't express what they want or what they feel through mimicry or looking; 4.Facial immobility

VIII. SLEEP DISORDERS

When they are small, they sleep many hours, and when they are older, they sleep few hours compared to the standard expected for their age. This behaviour may or may not be constant.

1. Doesn't want to go to sleep; 2. Gets up very early; 3. Sleeps irregularly (in intervals);
4. exchanges day for night; õ.sleeps very few hours.

IX. CHANGE IN DIET

It can be quantitative and/or qualitative. It can include situations from when the child stops eating to when they actively oppose it.

1 . Rigid food selectivity (e.g. always eating the same type of food);
2 Eating things other than food (paper, insects); 3. When he was small, he didn't

chew; 4. He has a ruminating activity; 5. He vomits; 6. He eats roughly, scatters food or throws it; 7. Rituals (crumbles food before eating); 8. Absence of taste (lack of taste sensitivity)

X. DIFFICULTY CONTROLLING SPHINCTERS

Sphincter control may exist, but its use can be a way of manipulating or attracting the adult's attention.

1. afraid to sit on the toilet; 2. uses the sphincters to manipulate the adult; 3. uses the sphincters as bodily stimulation, to obtain pleasure; 4. has daytime control, but nocturnal control is late or absent

XI. EXPLORING OBJECTS (TOUCHING, SUCKING)

Analyses objects sensorially, using the other sense organs more than sight, but without a specific purpose

1. Bites and swallows non-food objects; 2. Sucks and puts things in his mouth; 3. Smells everything; 4. Feels everything. Examines surfaces with their fingers in a meticulous manner

XII. INAPPROPRIATE USE OF OBJECTS

He doesn't use objects functionally, but in a bizarre way.

1. Ignores objects or shows momentary interest; 2.Picks up, hits or simply throws them on the floor; 3.Atypical behaviour with objects (holds indifferently in hands or spins); 4.Carries an object around insistently; 5.Is only interested in one part of the object or toy; 6.Collects strange objects; 7.Uses objects in a particular and inappropriate way

XIII. LACK OF ATTENTION

Difficulties with fixation and concentration. Sometimes fixes attention on their own sound or motor productions, giving the impression that they are absent.

1. When carrying out an activity, they fix their attention for a short time or are unable

to fix it; 2.They act as if they are deaf; 3.The response latency time is increased; 4.They understand instructions with difficulty (when they don't care, they don't understand them); õ.Delayed response; 6.They often give the feeling of absence

XIV. LACK OF INTEREST IN LEARNING

They have no interest in learning and seek solutions from others. Learning represents an effort of attention and personal exchange, it's a break in their routine.

1. Doesn't want to learn; 2. Gets tired very quickly, even in an activity they enjoy; 3. Forgets quickly; 4. Insists on being helped, even if they know how to do it; 5. Constantly insists on changing activities

XV. LACK OF INITIATIVE

Constantly seeks comfort and waits for everything to be handed to them. They don't carry out any functional activities on their own initiative.

1. Unable to take their own initiative; 2. Seeks comfort; 3. Passivity, lack of interest; 4. Slowness; õ.Prefers someone else to do the work for them

XVI. LANGUAGE AND COMMUNICATION DISORDERS

It is a fundamental characteristic of autism, which can range from a language delay to more severe forms, with exclusive use of particular and strange speech.

1. Mutism; 2. Vocal stereotypes; 3. Incorrect intonation; 4 Immediate and/or delayed echolalia; 5. Repetition of words or phrases that may or may not have communicative value; 6. Emits stereotyped sounds when agitated and at other times, for no apparent reason; 7. Does not communicate by gesture; 8. Interactions with an adult are never a dialogue

XVII. DOES NOT SHOW SKILLS AND KNOWLEDGE

They never express everything they are capable of doing or acting upon in terms of their knowledge and skills, making it difficult for professionals to assess them.

1. Even if they know how to do something, they don't do it if they don't want to; 2. They don't demonstrate what they know until they have a primary need or an imminently specific interest; 3. They learn things, but only demonstrate them in

certain places and with certain people; 4. They are sometimes surprised by their unexpected abilities

XVIII. INAPPROPRIATE REACTIONS TO FRUSTRATION

It ranges from annoyance to anger at frustration.

1. Reactions of displeasure if something is forgotten; 2.Reactions of displeasure if an activity they enjoy is interrupted; 3.Displeasure when wishes and expectations are not fulfilled; 4.Tantrum reactions

XIX. DOESN'T TAKE RESPONSIBILITY

In principle, it is incapable of taking responsibility, needing successive orders to do something.

1. Doesn't take on any responsibility, no matter how small; 2. In order to get anything done, they have to repeat themselves many times or raise their voice.

XX. HYPERACTIVITY/HYPOACTIVITY

The child can display anything from agitation, disorganised and uncontrolled excitement, to great passivity, with a total lack of response. These behaviours have no purpose.

1. The child is constantly on the move; 2. Even when stimulated, they don't move; 3. Noisy. Gives the feeling of being forced to make noise;

4. goes from one place to another without stopping; 5. keeps jumping in the same place; 6. never moves from where they are sitting

XXI. STEREOTYPED AND REPETITIVE MOVEMENTS

They occur in situations of rest or activity, with a sudden onset.

1. Swings; 2. Looks at and plays with hands and fingers; 3. Covers eyes and ears; 4. Kicks; 5. Makes faces and strange movements with the face; 6. Spins objects or on himself; 7. Walks on tiptoe or jumps, drags his feet, walks with strange movements; 8. Twists the body, maintains an unbalanced posture, legs bent, head collected at the feet, violent extensions of the body

XXII. IGNORES THE DANGER

You expose yourself without realising the danger

1 Doesn't realise the danger; 2. Climbs everywhere;

3. seems insensitive to pain

XXIII. **ONSET BEFORE 36 MONTHS (DSM-IV)**

Para cada item, escolha a coluna que melhor descreve o (a) aluno (a) (MARQUE UM X):

	Nem um pouco	Só um pouco	Bastante	Demais
1. Não consegue prestar muita atenção a detalhes ou comete erros por descuido nos trabalhos da escola ou tarefas				
2. Tem dificuldade de manter a atenção em tarefas ou atividades de lazer				
3. Parece não estar ouvindo quando se fala diretamente com ele				
4. Não segue instruções até o fim e não termina deveres de escola, tarefas ou obrigações.				
5. Tem dificuldade para organizar tarefas e atividades				
6. Evita, não gosta ou se envolve contra a vontade em tarefas que exigem esforço mental prolongado				
7. Perde coisas necessárias para atividades (ex: brinquedos, deveres da escola, lápis ou livros)				
8. Distrai-se com estímulos externos				
9. É esquecido em atividades do dia-a-dia				
10. Mexe com as mãos ou os pés ou se remexe na cadeira				
11. Sai do lugar na sala de aula ou em outras situações em que se espera que fique sentado				
12. Corre de um lado para outro ou sobe demais nas coisas em situações em que isto é inapropriado				
13. Tem dificuldade em brincar ou envolver-se em atividades de lazer de forma calma				
14. Não para ou frequentemente está a "mil por hora"				
15. Fala em excesso				
16. Responde as perguntas de forma precipitada antes delas terem sido terminadas				
17. Tem dificuldade de esperar sua vez				
18. Interrompe os outros ou se intromete (por exemplo: intromete-se nas conversas, jogos, etc.)				

ANNEX D - C-GAS: GLOBAL ASSESSMENT SCALE FOR CHILDREN AND ADOLESCENTS (04 TO 16 YEARS) - (Shaffer et al., 1983)

SPECIFIED TIME PERIOD: 1 MONTH

100 - 91 *Superior functioning* in all areas (at home, at school and with peers); involved in a large number of activities and has many interests (e.g. has "hobbies", or takes part in extracurricular activities, or belongs to an organised group such as the Scouts); sociable (pleasant), confident; everyday worries never get him down; does well at school; no symptoms.

90 - 81 *Functioning well in all areas;* stable in the family, at school and with peers; there may be transitory difficulties and (everyday) worries that occasionally get out of hand (e.g. slight anxiety associated with an important exam; occasional "outbursts" with siblings, parents or peers).

80 -71 *No more than a slight impairment in functioning* at home, at school or with peers; some behavioural problems or emotional overload may be present in response to life stressors (e.g. separation from parents; deaths; birth of a sibling), but these disturbances are brief and the interference with functioning is transitory; such children disturb others minimally and are not considered different from normal by those who know them.

70 - 61 *Some difficulty in a single area, but generally functions very well* (e g isolated or sporadic antisocial acts, such as occasionally carrying out petty theft; minor consistent or lasting difficulties with school work, short-lived mood swings, fears and anxieties that don't lead to overt avoidance behaviour, insecurity); has some meaningful interpersonal relationships; most people who don't know the child well wouldn't consider them problematic, but those who do know them express concern.

60 - 51 *Variable functioning with sporadic difficulties or symptoms in several but not all social areas;* disturbances are noticeable to those who meet the child at a dysfunctional time or *in* a dysfunctional environment, but not to those who see them at other times or *in* other environments.

50 - 41 *Moderate degree of interference in functioning in most social areas or severe* *dysfunction in a single area,* such as that which may result from, for example, suicidal ideation or ruminations, refusal to go to school and other forms of anxiety, obsessive rituals, major conversion symptoms, frequent anxiety attacks, impoverished or inappropriate social skills, frequent episodes of aggression or other antisocial behaviour, with some preservation of meaningful social relationships.

40 - 31 *Significant dysfunction in several areas and functional impairment in one of these areas: i.e.* maladaptive at home, at school, with peers or in society, e.g. persistent unprovoked aggression, marked apathy and isolation due to either mood or thought changes; suicidal attempts with clear lethal intent; usually such children require special schooling and/or hospitalisation or dismissal from school (but this is not a sufficient criterion for inclusion in this category).

30 - 21 *Functional incapacity in almost all areas,* e.g. staying at home, in the ward or in bed all day, not taking part in social activities or serious impairment in carrying out tests or serious impairment in communication (e.g. sometimes incoherent or inappropriate).

20 -11 *Needs considerable supervision* to prevent harm to others
or oneself (e.g. frequently violent, several suicide attempts) *or* to maintain personal hygiene *or* severe impairment in all forms of communication, e.g. severe abnormalities in verbal and gestural communication, severe social inadequacy, stupor, etc.

10-1 *Needs constant supervision* (24-hour care) due to intense aggression or self-destructive behaviour or severe impairment in performing tests, communication, cognition, affection or personal hygiene.

ANNEX E - VINELAND ADAPTIVE BEHAVIOUR SCALES^ (Sparrow SS et al., 1984)

Initials:________

RG-IP:- Date of birth: ________ //

Date: ____ //

COMMUNICATION DOMAIN

SCORING OF ITEMS:		
2	Yes, often.	A: Receptive
1	Sometimes or partially.	E: Expressive
0	No, never.	W: Writing
N	He didn't get the chance.	
DK	You don't know.	

		R	E	W
<1	1. Direct your gaze and head towards a sound.	( )		
	2. Pays attention at least momentarily when the carer speaks to them.	( )		
	3. Smiles at the presence of the carer.		( )	
	4. Smiles in the presence of a familiar person other than the carer.		( )	
	5. Raises his arms when the carer says: "Come here" or "Stand up".	( )		
	6. Demonstrates an understanding of the meaning of "no".	( )		
	7. Imitates adult sounds immediately after hearing them.		( )	
	8. Can understand the meaning of at least 10 words.	( )		
1	9. Can indicate "yes", "no" and "I want" appropriately with gestures.		( )	
	10. Listen carefully to commands.	( )		
	11. Understands the meaning of "yes" and "okay".	( )		
	12. Follows orders that require an action and an object.	( )		
	13. Correctly points to at least one main part of the body when questioned.	( )		
	14. Uses the first names or nicknames of siblings, friends or colleagues, or answers to their names when questioned.		( )	
	15. Uses sentences containing a noun and a verb, or two nouns.		( )	
	16. Name at least 20 familiar objects without being asked. DON'T POINT 1.		( )	
	17. Listen to a story for at least 5 minutes.	( )		
	18. Indicates preference when subjected to a choice.		( )	
2	19. Say at least 50 comprehensible words. DON'T POINT 1.		( )	
	20. Spontaneously reports experiences in simple language.		( )	
	21. Give a simple message.		( )	
	22. Uses sentences of 4 or more words.		( )	
	23. Points correctly to all parts of the body when questioned. DON'T POINT 1.	( )		
	24. Say at least 100 comprehensible words. DON'T POINT 1.		( )	
	25. Uses complete sentences.		( )	
	26. Use "a" and "the" in sentences.		( )	
	27. Follows orders in the "if/then" form.	( )		
	28. Tells his name and surname when questioned.		( )	
	29. Asks questions using "What", "Where", "Who", "Why" and "When". DON'T POINT 1.		( )	
3,4	30. Say which of two objects is bigger without them being present.		( )	
	31. Recounts experiences in detail when questioned.		( )	
	32. Use "behind" or "between" as a preposition in a sentence.		( )	
	33. Use "around" as a preposition in a sentence.		( )	
	34. Uses sentences containing "but" and "or".		( )	
	35. Articulates words clearly, without changing phonemes.		( )	
	36. Tells popular stories, fairy tales, longer jokes or extracts from television programmes.		( )	
5	37. Names all the letters of the alphabet from memory.			( )

		R	E	W
	38. Read at least three common signs.			( )
	39. Tells the day and month of his birthday when questioned.		( )	
	40. Uses irregular plurals.		( )	
6	41. Draws or writes their own name and surname.			( )
	42. Gives his telephone number when questioned. N CAN BE PUNCTUATED.		( )	
	43. Give your full address, including city and state, when questioned.		( )	
	44. Reads at least 10 words aloud or silently.			( )
	45. Draw or write at least 10 words from memory.			( )
	46. Expresses their ideas in more than one way, without help.		( )	
	47. Reads simple stories aloud.			( )
7,8	48. Draws or writes simple sentences of 3 or 4 words.			( )
	49. Attends a lesson for at least 15 minutes.	( )		
	50. Reads on own initiative.			( )
	51. Reads books from at least grade 2 .[a]			( )
	52. Sorts items or words alphabetically by first letter.			( )
	53. Draw or write little notes or messages.			( )
9	54. Explains complex itineraries to others.		( )	
	55. Writes rudimentary letters. DON'T POINT 1.			( )
	56. Reads books from at least grade 4 .[a]			( )
	57. Writes in handwriting most of the time. DON'T POINT 1.			( )
10 a 18+	58. Use a dictionary.			( )
	59. Uses the content relationship in reading material.			( )
	60. Write reports or essays. DON'T POINT 1.			( )
	61. Addresses envelopes correctly.			( )
	62. Use the index in reading material.			( )
	63. Reads stories from adult newspapers. N CAN BE SCORED.			( )
	64. It has realistic long-term objectives and describes in detail the strategies for achieving them.		( )	
	65. Writes elaborate letters.			( )
	66. Reads adult newspapers or weekly magazines. N CAN BE SCORED.			( )
	67. Write business letters. DON'T POINT 1.			( )

1.				SOMA:
2.				N°N:
3.				N°DK:
	R	E	W	Overall subdomain score:

ACTIVITIES OF COHDIAN LIFE DOMAIN

SCORING OF ITEMS:	
2 Yes, often.	Q: Guys
1 Sometimes or partially.	D: Domestic
0 No, never.	C: Community
N He didn't get the chance.	
DK You don't know.	

		P	D	C
<1	1. Shows awareness of the arrival of a bottle, breast or food.	( )		
	2. Open your mouth in front of the spoonful of food.	( )		
	3. Remove the food from the spoon with your mouth.	( )		
	4. Swallow or chew biscuits.	( )		
	5. Eat solid food.	( )		
1	6. Drinks from a cup or glass without assistance.	( )		
	7. Eats with a spoon.	( )		
	8. Demonstrates an understanding that hot things are dangerous.			( )
	9. Indicates that it is wet by pointing, talking or pulling on the nappy.	( )		
	10. Drink through a straw.	( )		
	11. Allows the carer to wipe their nose.	( )		
	12. Eats with a fork.	( )		
	13. Take off jacket with front opening, jumper or T-shirt without help.	( )		
2	14. Spoon-feeds without spilling.	( )		
	15. Shows an interest in changing when very wet or dirty.	( )		
	16. Urinating in the loo or toilet.	( )		
	17. Takes a bath without assistance.	( )		
	18. Flush down the loo or toilet.	( )		
	19. Asks to use the toilet.	( )		
	20. Fits removable clothes with adjustment straps.	( )		
	21. Demonstrates an understanding of the function of money.			( )
	22. Get rid of your possessions on request.		( )	
3	23. He doesn't urinate on his clothes at night.	( )		
	24. Drinks tap water without assistance.	( )		
	25. Brush your teeth without help. DON'T POINT 1.	( )		
	26. Demonstrates an understanding of the function of a clock, whether conventional or digital.			( )
	27. Helps with more tasks if asked.		( )	
	28. Washes and wipes face without assistance.	( )		
	29. Put the shoes on the correct feet without help.	( )		
	30. Answer the phone properly. CANNOT BE SCORED.			( )
	31. Dresses completely, except for tying shoes.	( )		
4	32. Calls the requested person on the phone or notifies them that they are not there. N CAN BE SCORED.			( )
	33. Sets the dining table without assistance.		( )	
	34. Takes all the necessary steps when going to the toilet, without needing to be reminded and without assistance. DON'T POINT 1.	( )		
	35. Look both ways before crossing the street or avenue.			( )
	36. Takes off clean clothes without assistance when asked.		( )	
	37. wipe your nose unaided. DON'T POINT 1.	( )		
	38. Clears table of fragile objects.		( )	
	39. wipes himself with a towel without help.	( )		
	40. Close all the zips. DO NOT POINT 1.	( )		
5	41. Helps prepare food that needs mixing and cooking		( )	

	42. Understands that it is dangerous to accept a lift, food or money from strangers.			( )
	43. Loops shoe laces without assistance.	( )		
	44. Takes a shower without assistance. DON'T POINT 1.	( )		
	45. Looks both ways and crosses the street or avenue alone.			( )
	46. Covers mouth and nose when coughing or sneezing.	( )		
6	47. Use spoon, fork and knife correctly. DON'T POINT 1.	( )		
	48. Initiates telephone calls to others. CANNOT BE SCORED.			( )
	49. Obeys traffic signs and "Stop" and "Walk" signals. CANNOT BE SCORED.			( )
	50. Dresses completely, including tying shoes and fastening zips. DON'T POINT 1.	( )		
	51. Tidies your bed when requested.		( )	
	52. Says the day of the week when asked.			( )
	53. Adjusts seat belt without help. N CAN BE SCORED.			( )
7	54. You know the value of each coin.			( )
	55. Use basic tools.		( )	
	56. Identifies right and left in others.			( )
	57. Tidies up the table without assistance when asked.		( )	
8	58. Sweeps, mops or hoovers carefully, without assistance, when requested.		( )	
	59. Use emergency telephone numbers in emergencies. N CAN BE SCORED.			( )
	60. Order your own dish in a restaurant. N CAN BE SCORED.			( )
	61. Says today's date if questioned.			( )
	62. Dresses in anticipation of changes in the weather without needing to be warned.	( )		
	63. Avoid people with contagious diseases, without having to be warned.	( )		
9, 10	64. Speak the time at 5-minute intervals.			( )
	65. Takes care of your hair without needing to be reminded and without help. DON'T POINT 1.	( )		
	66. Uses a cooker or microwave oven for cooking.		( )	
	67. Uses household cleaning products properly and correctly.		( )	
11, 12	68. Correctly give change for a purchase that costs more than one real.			( )
	69. Uses the telephone for all types of calls, without assistance. N CAN BE SCORED.			( )
	70. Cares for your nails without help and without having to be warned. DON'T POINT 1.	( )		
	71. Prepares food that needs mixing and cooking, without assistance.		( )	
13, 14, 15	72. Use a public telephone. CANNOT BE SCORED.			( )
	73. Tidy your room without needing to be reminded.		( )	
	74. Save up and buy at least one toy.			( )
	75. Take care of your own health.	( )		
16	76. Gets pocket money regularly.			( )
	77. You make your bed and change the sheets routinely. DON'T POINT 1.		( )	
	78. Cleans rooms other than his own regularly, without		( )	

	prompting.				
	79. Carries out routine household maintenance and repairs without prompting.		( )		
17 a 18+	80. Sews buttons, buttonholes and hooks onto clothes when required.		( )		
	81. Budgets for monthly expenses.				( )
	82. He takes care of his money without help.				( )
	83. Plans and prepares the main course of the day without assistance.		( )		
	84. He gets to work on time.				( )
	85. Takes care of your clothes without needing to be reminded. DON'T POINT 1.		( )		
	86. Notify your supervisor if you're going to be late.				( )
	87. Notify your supervisor if you are going to be absent due to illness.				( )
	88. Budgets for monthly expenses.				( )
	89. He makes his own hems and other alterations without having to be warned.		( )		
	90. Obeys time limits for coffee and lunch at work.				( )
	91. takes on full-time work with responsibility. DON'T POINT 1.				( )
	92. He has a bank account and handles it responsibly.				( )

1.				SOMA:
2.				N°N:
3.				N°DK:
	P	D	C	Overall subdomain score:

SOCIALISATION DOMAIN

SCORING OF ITEMS:	
2Yes , often.	IR: Interpersonal Relations PLT: Play and
1Sometimes or partially.	Leisure CS: Social Skills
0No , never.	
He didn't get the chance.	
DKDon't know.	

		IR	PLT	CS
<1	1. Look at the carer's face.	( )		
	2. Reacts to the voice of the carer or another person.	( )		
	3. Distinguish the carer from others.	( )		
	4. Shows interest in new objects or people.		( )	
	5. Expresses two or more understandable emotions such as pleasure, sadness, fear or distress.	( )		
	6. Anticipates being picked up by the carer.	( )		
	7. Shows affection towards family members.	( )		
	8. Shows interest in children other than their siblings.		( )	

	9. You're addressing someone you know.	( )		
	10. Plays with a toy or other object alone or accompanied.		( )	
	11. Participates in simple interactive games with other children.		( )	
	12. Uses household objects to play with.		( )	
	13. Shows interest in the activities of others.		( )	
	14. Imitates simple adult movements, such as clapping or waving goodbye, in response to a model.	( )		
1,2	15. Laughs and smiles appropriately in response to positive stimuli.	( )		
	16. Identifies at least two family members by name.	( )		
	17. shows a desire to please the carer.	( )		
	18. Participates in at least one group activity or game.		( )	
	19. Imitates a relatively complex task several hours after it has been performed by someone else.	( )		
	20. Imitates adult phrases heard on previous occasions.	( )		
	21. Strives to create "make-believe" situations, alone or with others.		( )	
3	22. shows preference for some friends over others.	( )		
	23. Say "Please" when asking for something.			( )
	24. Qualifies happiness, sadness, fear and anger in itself.	( )		
	25. Identifies people by characteristics other than their name, when asked.	( )		
4	26. Shares toys and objects without needing to request.		( )	
	27. Name one or more favourite television programmes when asked, and say on which days and channels the programmes are shown. N CAN BE SCORED.		( )	
	28. Follows rules in simple games without needing to be reminded.		( )	
	29. Has a favourite friend of any gender.	( )		
	30. Follows school rules and routines.			( )
5	31. reacts verbally and positively to the good results of others.	( )		
	32. Ask for forgiveness for unintentional mistakes.			( )
	33. You have a group of friends.	( )		
	34. Follow the community rules.			( )
6	35. Plays more than one table game or card game that requires skill and decision.		( )	
	36. Don't talk with your mouth full.			( )
	37. Has a bosom friend of the same sex.	( )		
	38. Reacts appropriately when introduced to someone.			( )
7,8	39. Makes or buys small gifts for the carer or family member on festive dates, on their own initiative.	( )		
	40. Keeps secrets and confidences for more than a day.			( )
	41. Returns toys, objects or money borrowed from a classmate and returns books borrowed from the library.			( )
	42. End the conversation properly.			( )
9	43. Follows time limits imposed by the carer.			( )

		IR	PLT	CS
	44. Avoid questions or comments that could embarrass or hurt others.			( )
	45. Controls anger and hurt when denied.			( )
	46. Keep secrets and confidences as much as is appropriate.			( )
10, 11	47. Behaves appropriately at the table without needing to be warned. DON'T POINT 1.			( )
	48. Watches TV or listens to the radio in search of information about a particular area of interest. N CAN BE SCORED.		( )	
	49. Goes to night school or closed events with friends, when accompanied by an adult. N CAN BE SCORED.		( )	
	50. They weigh up the consequences of their actions before making independent decisions.			( )
	51. Ask forgiveness for errors in judgement.			( )
12, 13, 14	52. Remembers birthdays of close family members and friends in particular.	( )		
	53. Initiates conversations on topics of special interest to others.	( )		
	54. You have a hobby.		( )	
	55. Returns money borrowed from the carer.			( )
15 a 18+	56. Reacts to allusions and hints during conversation.	( )		
	57. Participates in extracurricular sports. CANNOT BE SCORED.		( )	
	58. Watches TV or listens to the radio for practical, everyday information. N CAN BE SCORED.		( )	
	59. Schedules and respects appointments.			( )
	60. Watches TV or listens to the radio independently looking for news. N CAN BE SCORED.		( )	
	61. Goes to night school or closed events with friends, unaccompanied by an adult. N CAN BE SCORED.		( )	
	62. Goes out at night with friends without adult supervision.		( )	
	63. Belongs to a social or service organisation, interest group or organised club of older teenagers.	( )		
	64. Going with a single person of the opposite sex to parties or public events where many people will be present.	( )		
	65. I go out in groups of two or three couples.	( )		
	66. Go out on dates alone.	( )		

1.				SOMA:
2.				N°N:
3.				N°DK:
	IR	PLT	CS	Overall subdomain score:

MOTOR SKILLS DOMAIN

SCORING OF ITEMS:	
2 Yes , often.	G: Coarse
1 Sometimes or partially.	F: Fine
0 No, never.	
N He didn't get the chance.	
DK You don't know.	

		G	F
<1	1. holds the head upright for at least 15 seconds unaided when supported vertically by the examiner's arms.	( )	
	2. Sit with support for at least 1 minute.	( )	
	3. Grasps small objects with his hands in any way.		( )
	4. Transfers objects from one hand to the other.		( )
	5. Grasps small objects with thumb and fingers.		( )
	6. Rise to a sitting position and hold the position for at least 1 minute.	( )	
	7. Crawls across the floor on hands and knees, without touching their belly to the floor.	( )	
	8. Opens doors that only need to be pushed or pulled.		( )
1	9. Roll a ball while sitting down.	( )	
	10. You walk with the aim of exploring your surroundings.	( )	
	11. Gets up and down from the bed or a large chair.	( )	
	12. Climb on low toys.	( )	
	13. Scribbles with pencil, crayon or chalk on surfaces.		( )
2	14. Climb stairs with both feet on each step.	( )	
	15. Go down the stairs facing forwards, with both feet on each step.	( )	
	16. Runs gracefully, with changes of speed and direction.	( )	
	17. Opens doors by turning and pushing handles.		( )
	18. Jumps over small objects.	( )	
	19. Screw on and unscrew the lid of a pot.		( )
	20. Pedals a tricycle or other three-wheeled vehicle for at least three feet. N CAN BE SCORED.	( )	
	21. Standing on one foot while holding onto another person or stable object without falling.	( )	
	22. Build structures in three dimensions with at least 5 blocks.		( )
	23. Open and close scissors with one hand.		( )
3, 4+	24. Descends stairs unaided, alternating feet.	( )	
	25. Climb on tall toys.	( )	
	26. Cut out paper with scissors.		( )
	27. Jump on one foot at least three times without losing momentum.	( )	
	DON'T POINT 1.		
	28. Complete a jigsaw puzzle with at least 6 pieces. DON'T POINT 1.		( )
	29. Draws more than one recognisable shape with pencil or crayon.		( )
	30. Cut out paper following a line with the scissors.		( )
	31. Use the eraser without tearing the paper.		( )
	32. Jumps on one foot with ease. DON'T POINT 1.	( )	
	33. Unlocks locks.		( )
	34. Cut out complex figures with scissors.		( )
	35. Catches a small ball thrown from a distance of 10 feet, even if he has to move to do so.	( )	
	36. Ride a bicycle without safety wheels without falling off. CANNOT BE SCORED.	( )	
		G	F

1.		**SOMA:**
2.		**N°N:**

3.			DK NO:
	G	F	Overall subdomain score:

DISRUPTIVE BEHAVIOUR DOMAIN

SCORING OF ITEMS:	
2	Yes, often.
1	Sometimes or partially.
0	No, never.
N	He didn't get the chance.
DK	You don't know.

PART 1

1. Sucks thumb or fingers.	( )
2. He's too dependent.	( )
3. Hide.	( )
4. Bedwetting.	( )
5. Has an eating disorder.	( )
6. Has a sleep disorder.	( )
7. Bite your nails.	( )
8. Avoids school or work.	( )
9. Shows marked anxiety.	( )
10. Has tics.	( )
11. Cries or laughs very easily.	( )
12. Has little eye contact.	( )
13. Excessive unhappiness.	( )
14. Range of teeth during the day or night.	( )
15. He's very impulsive.	( )
16. Poor ability to pay attention and concentrate.	( )
17. He's too active.	( )
18. He has tantrums.	( )
19. Negative or defiant.	( )
20. Torment or threaten.	( )
21. Shows a lack of consideration.	( )
22. Lies, cheats or steals.	( )
23. He's physically very aggressive.	( )
24. Yours in inappropriate situations.	( )
25. Run away.	( )
26. Stubborn or bad-tempered.	( )
27. Is a gazetteer at school or work.	( )

PART 2

INTENSITY

CIRCLE ONE OF THEM

		GRAVE	MODERATE
28. Engages in inappropriate sexual behaviour.	( )	S	M
29. Has excessive or peculiar preoccupations with objects or activities.	( )	S	M
30. Expresses thoughts that are not sensible.	( )	S	M

31. Demonstrates extremely peculiar mannerisms or habits.	( )	S	M
32. Engages in self-injurious behaviour.	( )	S	M
33. Intentionally destroys own or other people's property.	( )	S	M
34. Presents bizarre speech.	( )	S	M
35. He's oblivious to what's going on around him.	( )	S	M
36. Sways back and forth when sitting or standing.	( )	S	M

SOMA (PART 1 and 2):

ANNEX F - INFORMED CONSENT FORM

UNIVERSITY OF SÃO PAULO

INSTITUTE OF PSYCHOLOGY
DEVELOPMENTAL DISORDERS LABORATORY

Av. Professor Mello Moraes, 1721 - Bloco G, 2º andar, sala 27
CEP 05508-030 - Cidade Universitária - São Paulo/SP

Tel (11)3091-4182

CNS Resolution No. 466/2012, according to the National Health Council (CNS)

Available at

http://www.ip.usp.br/portal/index.php?option=com_content&view=article&id=312&Itemid

=283&lang=en

Dear person responsible for_______________________________________

(child's name)

The project "STUDY OF PSYCHIATRIC COMORBITIES IN CEREBRAL PARALYSIA" is being carried out by neuropediatrician Alessandra Freitas Russo, from USP's Developmental Disorders Laboratory and AACD - Osasco, located at Av. Getúlio Vargas 1150, Osasco, CEP 06233-20.

More detailed information about the project can be obtained by calling (11) 3604-5203 (Researcher) or by e-mailing arusso@usp.br.

Objective: To assess the presence of psychiatric disorders in children with cerebral palsy

Procedure: Screening scales for psychiatric disorders will be applied during a clinical assessment visit.

Benefits: The results will enable a better approach to the treatment of cerebral palsy.

Risk: There will be no risk to the physical (health) or moral integrity of the children. This assessment does not cause discomfort.

Privacy: The data will be confidential. The results will be collated and processed collectively. They may be published in scientific conferences and publications without the child's name. Your participation is voluntary. If you do not agree to take part in the research, there will be no impediment or changes in the relationship between you, your child and the AACD, and you may withdraw your consent and stop taking part in the research at any time, including before its end.

Signature of legal guardian   Researcher's signature

I.. (name of responsible),   responsible   for .... (child's name), I have been informed of the objectives of the research "STUDY OF PSYCHIATRIC COMORBITIES IN CEREBRAL PARALYSIS" above in a clear and detailed manner. I received information about the procedures and clarified any doubts I had. I know that at any time I can request new information and change my decision to allow my participation if I wish, without any kind of penalty. I have been assured that all data from this research will be kept confidential and that I will be free to withdraw my consent to take part in the research at any time.

Child's name: ....
Identity document: ....Date of birth:...................................Sex: M() F ()
Name of person in charge: ....
Nature (degree of kinship, guardian, carer, etc.):...
Identity Document:....................................Date of Birth: ....
Address:.. No.: .... Apt.:....CEP: ....
City:.. UF:.............. Telephone: (.)...................... Date: ....
Signature of legal guardian   Researcher's signature

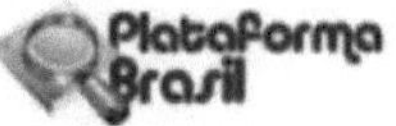

HOSPITAL E CENTRO DE REABILITAÇÃO DA AACD

PARECER CONSUBSTANCIADO DO CEP

Elaborado pela Instituição Coparticipante

DADOS DO PROJETO DE PESQUISA

Título da Pesquisa: COMORBIDADES PSIQUIATRICAS NA PARALISIA CEREBRAL
Pesquisador: ALESSANDRA FREITAS RUSSO
Área Temática:
Versão: 1
CAAE: 31130714.4.3001.0085
Instituição Proponente: UNIVERSIDADE DE SAO PAULO
Patrocinador Principal: Financiamento Próprio

DADOS DO PARECER

Número do Parecer: 1.007.076
Data da Relatoria: 26/01/2015

Apresentação do Projeto:
COMORBIDADES PSIQUIATRICAS NA PARALISIA CEREBRAL- somos instituição co participantes, pois este projeto já foi aprovado em primeira instância no CEP da instituição proponente

Objetivo da Pesquisa:
Pesquisar a prevalência de comorbidades psiquiátricas em crianças e adolescentes com paralisia cerebral atendidos em um centro de reabilitação terciário.

Avaliação dos Riscos e Benefícios:
foi incluido o termo risco mínimo conforme orientação anterior, pois o sujeito da pesquisa são crianças e adolescentes.

Comentários e Considerações sobre a Pesquisa:
pesquisa interessante que pode de fato abrir um leque maior para disgnósticos psiquiatricos diferencial. para crianças e adolescentes com paralisia cerebral

Considerações sobre os Termos de apresentação obrigatória:
sem considerações a serem feitas

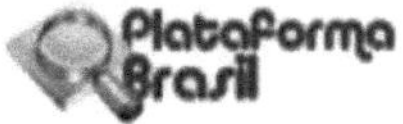

Continuação do Parecer: 1.007.076

*Rever a idade ou o testes que se propõe a utilizar pois a idade de 17a e 11 meses, nenhum dos testes psicológicos sugeridos atinge essa população

*Não encontrado um co autor da institução participante

Conclusões ou Pendências e Lista de Inadequações:

rever às recomendações acima sugeridas

Situação do Parecer:

Aprovado

Necessita Apreciação da CONEP:

Não

Considerações Finais a critério do CEP:

O Colegiado do CEP, reunido em plenária no dia 31 de março de 2015, reitera as observações da Relatoria: 1. Como o projeto está sendo realizado na Associação de Assistência à Criança Deficiente (na qualidade de co-participante), há uma normativa institucional da necessidade de um membro da AACD na qualidade de Colaborador do projeto e que deve, por extensão, constar na lista de autores por ocasião da publicação e; 2. Sugerimos ao autor que verifique a adequabilidade das escalas utilizadas em função das idades dos pacientes avaliados. O CEP encontra-se à disposição para dirimir eventuais dúvidas. Orientamos que nos seja enviado o(s) artigo(s) publicado(s) da tese já com a participação do membro da AACD. Além disso, gostaríamos de receber um exemplar da tese para que constasse em nossos bancos de dados.

SAO PAULO, 31 de Março de 2015

Assinado por:
Luis Garcia Alonso
(Coordenador)

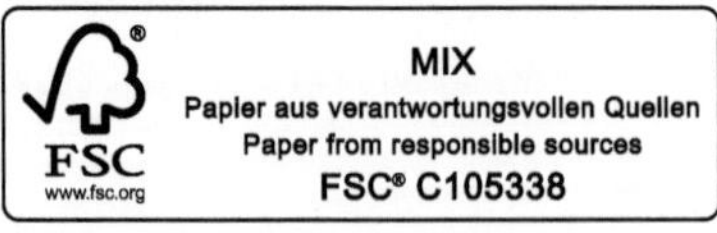

Printed by Books on Demand GmbH, Norderstedt / Germany